D0198004

This book is dedicated to my adorable sons,
Luca and Matteo. Your sweet smiles, cute
personalities, delicious kisses, and love for life have
become my inspiration for all that I do.
I am so lucky to be your mom. May God always
bless your hearts with faith, goodness, and health.

XOXO,
Your Mamma

8.00
(49).

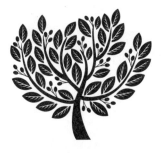

The Full-Fat Solution

Good Fats for a Lean Body, a Healthy Heart,
Smart Children, and Delicious Food

KARLENE KARST, R.D.

© 2016 Karlene Karst

All rights reserved.

Printed in Canada

This book may not be reproduced in whole or in part, in any form or by any means, electronic or mechanical, including photocopying, recording, or by any information storage and retrieval system now known or hereafter invented, without permission from the author.

Books are available for special promotions and premiums. For details, contact karlene@karlenekarst.com.

ISBN-13: 978-1-936961-09-2
ISBN-10: 1-936961-09-1
Library of Congress Control Number: 2012945366

Book Design by Jonathan Selikoff
Editing by Andrea Lemieux
Cover Photo by Tonino Guzzo

You should always consult with your doctor before making any changes to your diet, or starting an exercise program.

Contents

Acknowledgments

My career in the natural health industry has spanned over a decade. During this time, my life has been blessed with incredible richness, knowledge, health, a husband, children, and the opportunity to travel and see the world. My faith in Christ has served as the basis and the guiding factor in all the decisions I have made, both personally and professionally.

My husband, Gaetano, has been my biggest fan. When I chose him as my partner, I found a person who would not only support me personally, but also believed in me more than I even believe in myself and gave me the confidence to achieve what I once thought was impossible. Gaetano encouraged me to write this book and has been extremely patient and understanding with my early mornings, late nights, and ups and downs during the book-writing process. I would truly not be where I am today in all aspects of my life if it weren't for his incredible brilliance, passion, and perseverance. Our partnership and journey in life is only just beginning. Gaetano, thank you!

I have dedicated this book to my adorable sons, Luca and Matteo. These boys are the absolute light of my life. When it comes to health, they have been taking their liquid fish oil since they were six months old, along with vitamins and probiotics, and drinking protein shakes and making spinach and kale smoothies in the blender with me. They are full of life and love, and tears come to my eyes when I think of how much I love my boys. Thank you, Luca and Matteo, for the opportunity to parent you and be your mom. You make me so proud.

The Full-Fat Solution is a follow-up to the national best-selling book *Healthy Fats for Life*, which I coauthored with Lorna

Vanderhaeghe. I would like to acknowledge Lorna for the mentoring and friendship she has given me over the years.

There are many other people involved in writing and publishing a book. I thank my publisher, Steve Eunpu, and my editor, Andrea Lemieux, for their literary expertise. I am grateful to my entire family and numerous friends who have always encouraged me and been excited for me for all the opportunities that have come my way. And to my publicist, Rhoda Rizkalla-Couvaras, you are a gem of a friend, and I am so lucky to have you in my corner. I will never forget what you have done for me.

Many blessings for health and happiness!
Live with Health,

Karlene

Introduction

As a dietitian, I have seen many concepts about food and nutrition come full circle. Of all the nutrient categories, I believe that fats have been the most misunderstood, criticized, and challenged; however, they are now becoming an accepted and embraced nutrient group. When I was studying nutrition in the mid-1990s, fat was evil: saturated fat caused heart disease, coconut oil would increase your cholesterol, and butter would clog your arteries. I listened to this teaching with much interest, thinking to myself, "How can this be? My mom has been using butter in our cooking for the past twenty years." On weekends at home, I would let my mom know all about the bad things she was eating—and feeding us—such as whole milk and butter, to name just a few. As an adult, and mom, I give my boys organic whole milk; we also eat and cook certain foods with organic butter and coconut oil, among many other expeller-pressed oils, and we eat full-fat Greek yogurt and avocados often, and, luckily, my boys have been drinking fish oil from the bottle since they were six months old. Yes, thankfully, it seems that fat has come full circle.

Since the 1980s, low-fat and no-fat foods with dangerous trans fats (those hidden phantom fats) have lined our grocery-store shelves—oh yes, they still do! Everything from low-fat cookies to low-fat salad dressings carry the message that we can lose weight and get healthy by cutting out or reducing fat in our diets. Yet, while the focus was on reducing fat, little did we know that the real nutrition evil was the excess sugar in the food we were eating, and we saw skyrocketing rates of obesity, type-2 diabetes, heart disease, metabolic syndrome, and cancer.

Chronic diseases of inadequate nutrition affect up to 80 percent of North Americans. We are the most overfed, undernourished continent in the world, filling our bodies with empty calories and toxic foods with very dangerous side effects.

A decade ago, I was encouraging clients to get back to the basics of nutrition and return to a diet consisting of whole foods; fresh, organically grown fruit and vegetables; wild fish; free-range chicken and eggs; grass-fed beef; nuts and seeds; and whole grains. And, of course, healthful real fat from dark green leafy vegetables, expeller-cold-pressed oils from flaxseed and grapeseed, avocados, butter, coconut oil, full-fat dairy products, and the list goes on.

Consumers across North America consistently ask me about what oils to buy, how to store them, how to cook with them, and, above all, what they are supposed to be eating. I encourage everyone to not only get back to the basics and eat real food but also to start cooking again. I know we are all busy. My husband and I both work more than full time, running our business and traveling to give lectures and interviews, and we have two adorable sons, Luca and Matteo, among many other obligations. Are we able to cook from scratch every night? The honest answer is no. But are we able to cook real food more often than not? The answer to this is a resounding yes. We need to cook again, we need to sit down as a family and enjoy our food and meals. Food is not only fuel for our bodies, but it provides enjoyment, opportunities for communication, and a sense of family as well. Involve your kids in the process; they will *love* it. Use Sunday evening to plan what to make for dinner on three of the five work nights of the week, and, of course, make enough for leftovers for the following night.

My goal with *The Full-Fat Solution* is to ensure that you and your families are eating the best food—and fat—possible. Long gone are the days of avoiding fat; we need to embrace it. Fat is essential, and healthful fats are a must for reaching your optimal health. Extensive scientific research has validated the benefits of healthful fats for glowing skin, shiny hair, strong nails, flexible joints, balanced hormones, a lean body, a healthy heart, and smart children. Within four weeks of incorporating healthful fats into each of your meals and snacks, the benefits to your health will shine from within.

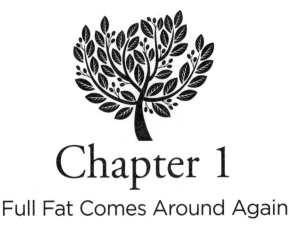

Chapter 1

Full Fat Comes Around Again

We have come full circle with the nutrient fat, from full fat to low fat, and now to focusing again on healthful, full-fat foods in our diet as a way to ensure optimal health, energy, and a balanced body. We know that a lack of certain fats in the diet can be detrimental to our health. Not to mention that most people who begin to reduce their fat intake will eat more high-carbohydrate items, such as pasta, muffins, breads, and sugary foods. Instead of seeing a decrease in diabetes, heart disease, and weight gain, we have witnessed an unprecedented increase in these conditions.

The focus of this chapter is to provide an overview of the different fats and the science behind them.

Years Ago

Major changes in the type and amount of fat we consume have occurred over the past forty to fifty years, as reflected in increases in saturated fat (from animal sources and hydrogenated oils), trans fats, vegetables oils rich in omega-6 fatty acids, and an overall decrease in the omega-3s.

Ancient food records reveal diets that consisted mainly of wild meat, fish, plants, nuts, seeds, and berries. Grains and sugars were absent from human nutrition until the development of agriculture 10,000 years ago. Moving forward to the present day, the reliance on grocers to provide food, and the grocers' financial concern to keep wasted food down to a minimum, paved the way for the highly processed and preserved foodstuffs we find in our supermarkets today.

Build Your Cells from Fat: Healthful Fat, That Is

There are some fats that are necessary for the body to function, and you should include them in your diet. However, there are other fats that can kill you, and most of us are eating them every day. Bad fats are associated with cancer, heart disease, diabetes, and arthritis, but good fats can reduce inflammation, burn unwanted fat, stabilize blood sugar levels, and lower blood pressure. It is important to understand which fats you should be leaving out of your meals and which should be going in.

There are two main groups of fats—saturated and unsaturated.

1. Saturated Fats
The Very Good, the Good, the Bad, and the Ugly

Saturated fats are semisolid at room temperature and are found in animal products, such as red meat, pork, lamb, lard, and dairy products, such as milk, cheese, and butter, as well as in processed foods. They have been generally considered "bad" fats as research once showed a link to heart disease; therefore, especially in the past, nutritional researchers and health officials have recommended a reduction of saturated fats in the diet. Contrary to popular belief, full-fat dairy, including milk, butter, and cheese, has never been convincingly linked to cardiovascular disease.

However, I have some great news to share, not all saturated fats are created equally. Saturated fats are actually useful for energy production, satiety, and hormones. We are much more sophisticated in our knowledge of saturated fats, so don't be too quick to get rid of your butter, coconut oil, and full-fat dairy in place of lower saturated fat alternatives. In fact, in my house we favor full-fat dairy, such as rich, creamy Greek yogurt, whole milk, and full-fat sour cream. A little goes a long way as the full-fat varieties are much more satisfying to the palate and provide a feeling of satiety, not to mention they taste better. A new Australian study reports that eating full-fat dairy products could even prevent heart disease or strokes. Scientists from the Queensland Institute of Medical Research surveyed 1,500 people on their eating habits for a period of sixteen years. They found those who had the highest intake of full-fat dairy had a 70 percent lower risk of death from heart disease or stroke. The lead researcher, Dr. Joleike van der Pols, says there may be some nutrients in full-fat dairy products that counteract any negative effects of saturated fat.[1] A study from the Harvard School of Public Health suggests that in the case of dairy products, full-fat dairy may have benefits and reduce your risk of diabetes. But interestingly, it wasn't the fat as much as the trans-palmitoleic acid in the bloodstream that seemed to provide the protective benefit. This study included more than 3,700 adults age sixty-five and older. The people who reported eating more full-fat dairy had higher levels of trans-palmitoleic acid in their bloodstream. Other benefits related to this included less body fat, higher HDL cholesterol, lower C-reactive protein, and lower triglyceride levels. They also showed a 60 percent lower incidence of diabetes.[2]

I expand on the intriguing topic of full-fat dairy in chapter 2.

Allow me to explain saturated fats further. The three subgroups of saturated fats are based on their fat-chain length: short-chain, medium-chain, and long-chain. And then there are trans fats, the artificially saturated fats.

The Very Good: Short-Chain Saturated Fats

Short-chain saturates, found in butter, coconut oil, and palm kernel oil do not clog arteries, nor do they cause heart disease. Rather, they are easily digested and a source of fuel for energy. As well, short-chain saturates do not contain as many calories as the longer-chain fatty acids. Butter is only 80 percent fat, and margarine is 100 percent fat, so one pound of butter has eight fewer calories than a pound of margarine made with seed oils.

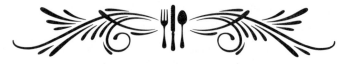

Better Butter

To make butter even better, mix ½ pound (250 g) of organic butter with ¼ cup (60 mL) of your favorite essential-fat oil (I especially favor organic flaxseed oil by Barlean's). This is excellent as a spread on sprouted-grain bread, a whole-wheat muffin, or any of your other favorite snacks. Store better butter in the refrigerator for ultimate freshness.

The Good: Medium-Chain Saturated Fats

Medium-chain saturates are found in several foods, but the highest content (just as in short-chain saturates) is found in palm kernel oil and coconut oil, and they are not associated with increased cholesterol levels or the occurrence of heart disease (which was at one time thought to be the case; however, when the science was investigated further, it was found that the lack of essential fats in the diet was the cause of heart disease). The properties of medium-chain fats found in plant sources such as coconut are different from those of animal origin. Medium-chain fats do not undergo degradation and re-esterification processes and are directly used in the body to produce energy. Medium-chain triglyceride (MCT) oils are also used in special nutritional formulas for people who need energy from fat but have trouble digesting it from regular dietary sources, and they are used by athletes looking to convert fat into energy rather than store it as fat.

The Bad: Long-Chain Saturated Fats

Long-chain saturates are the "bad" fats associated with raising LDL (the bad cholesterol), lowering HDL (the good cholesterol), and the increasing the risk of heart disease. The bad saturated fats are those primarily found in red meat. Long-chain saturates are also a by-product of hydrogenation, a process that turns a liquid fat (at room temperature) into a solid, as is employed in the manufacture of most margarines and shortenings. Long-chain saturates are also abundantly present in restaurant food, fried food, junk food, packaged baked goods, and processed food. Hydrogenation or partial hydrogenation also distorts the fatty acids into a more poisonous form.

The Ugly: Trans Fats

Trans fats are by far the worst type of fat. Numerous research studies have shown that trans fats are more damaging to the heart than saturated fats. The Institute of Medicine's dietary reference intakes report declared there is no safe level of trans fats and that consumption should be reduced as much as possible.[3]

Trans fats were developed when there was a backlash against saturated fats. They are artificial, formed by a process of high temperature and hydrogenation that turns refined oils into margarines, shortenings, and partially hydrogenated vegetable oils, making them solid or semisolid and "shelf stable." Our bodies cannot recognize them as nutrients and, therefore, are not able to process them. They are, however, a food manufacturer's dream as they are inexpensive to produce and extend the shelf life of foods.

Operation Covert Trans-Fatty Acids

As you shop for your usual grocery items, read the labels and add up the percentages of fat. There is a good chance they will not equal 100 percent. The missing percentage could be the poisonous trans fats.

2. Unsaturated Fats

Unsaturated fats are liquid at room temperature and are generally considered to be "good" fats. Typically, the more liquid a fat is, the more healthful it is. Unsaturated fats can be further classified as either a monounsaturated fatty acid (MUFA) or a polyunsaturated fatty acid (PUFA). MUFAs remain liquid at room temperature but solidify in colder temperatures. Sources of these are olive, canola, and macadamia nut oils. These fatty acids are associated with good cholesterol.

PUFAs remain liquid at room temperature and remain in liquid form even in colder temperatures. Sources of PUFAs include safflower, sunflower, and evening primrose oils; fatty fish; and dark green leafy vegetables, such as kale, broccoli, Brussels sprouts, and purslane, as well as an assortment of nuts and seeds, such as walnuts, almonds, macadamia nuts, hemp seeds, and flaxseeds. Dietary reference studies show that approximately 2 grams (0.07 oz.) of the omega-3 alpha-linoleic acid (LA) is consumed from a plant-based diet.

Unsaturated fats can be further classified into three major classes: omega-3, omega-6, and omega-9. The omega-3s and omega-6s are polyunsaturated, and they are called "essential" because the body cannot make them. The omega-9s are monounsaturated and "nonessential" because the body can make them from other fatty acids.

Understanding Essential Fatty Acids (EFAs): Why Essential Fats Are So Essential

Essential fatty acids are polyunsaturated fats that include the following:

- The omega-6 fatty acid alpha-linoleic acid (LA) and its metabolites gamma-linolenic acid (GLA) and arachidonic acid (AA).

- The omega-3 fatty acid alpha-linolenic acid (ALA) and its metabolites eicosapentaenoic acid (EPA) and docosahexaenoic acid (DHA).

Theoretically, only LA and ALA are absolutely essential. However, the fatty acids derived from them are also generally considered essential. Deficiencies in EFAs are common today for three reasons: (1) modern dietary and lifestyle choices, (2) the effects of environmental pollution, and (3) some people have trouble converting LA and ALA to their metabolites, which are responsible for hormone production.

The Functions of EFAs

The three main functions of EFAs are to regulate cellular processes, influence membrane function and integrity, and produce hormones that regulate and balance inflammation and immune responses.

1. Cell Processes

The cellular processes that fatty acids regulate include the following:

- Regulation of enzymes
- Regulation of cell signaling pathways
- Attachment of proteins to fatty acids
- Regulation of gene expression
- Gene activation
- Receptor function and activation
- Membrane permeability
- Ion channels (the transport system for potassium and sodium)
- Transport properties
- Oxidation of fats

- Communication from the cell membrane to the nucleus of the cell
- Lipid signaling

2. Cell Membrane Integrity

Cell Membranes made from EFAs

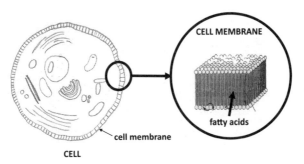

EFAs are integral components of cell membranes, determining fluidity and other physical properties as well as affecting structural functions; for example, the maintenance of enzyme activity. Our bodies are built of billions of cells. Cells are built of membranes, and membranes are built of fats. Cell membranes built with polyunsaturated essential fats are less rigid and more fluid than membranes built with saturated fats. Fluid cells are extremely important because they allow the transport of valuable nutrients into the cells, they help keep toxins out of the cells, they elasticize tissue, they expand blood vessel walls to reduce heart workload, and they improve the overall function of organs.

If your cells are built of saturated fats, they will become rigid and hard. You may not notice the effects of your diet and its role in health when you are young, but if you continue to consume a diet full of unhealthful fats, you will start to see the effects manifested in inflammatory conditions, such as arthritis, insulin resistance, metabolic syndrome, cardiovascular disease, and diabetes. It is extremely important that your cells are built from healthful fats, which keep the cells fluid. Fluid cells influence insulin sensitivity; they help your body utilize the insulin produced by your pancreas, and they help control your body's glucose levels.

3. The Power of Hormones

Early researchers believed that all the benefits of EFAs were attributed to their role in maintaining the cellular processes and the integrity and function of the cell membrane. It was decades later, in the early 1970s, when scientists learned the body also uses EFAs to produce a family of powerful hormone-like compounds. Some of the most potent effects of EFAs are related to their conversion into a series of eicosanoids, or hormones. They are intracellular communication agents that control the balance of virtually every system in the body, including the mechanisms for inflammation, blood clotting, and blood vessel dilation. They include, but are not limited to, anti-inflammatory and inflammatory prostaglandins (PGE series 1, 2, and 3) and other immune-system responders, such as thromboxanes, leukotrienes, and hydroxy fatty acids, and, recently, research has revealed a new class of mediators called "resolvins" and "protectins." Although humans and animals can synthesize saturated and monounsaturated fatty acids, they lack the enzymes needed to insert a cis double bond at the omega-3 or the omega-6 positions of a fatty acid to synthesize ALA or LA, respectively. These two fatty acids share a common metabolic pathway in which they compete for the delta-6-desaturase, the first step in the metabolism pathway.

The Metabolic Pathway for Omega-6 Linoleic Acid (LA)

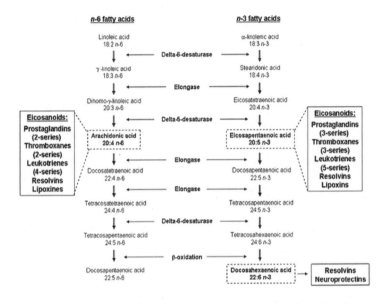

Under optimal conditions, the body processes linoleic acid, one of the two primary essential fatty acids needed for health, through a series of steps that eventually leads to the production of hormones. The omega-6 pathway shows how LA produces GLA with the help of the delta-6-desaturase enzyme, or D6D enzyme. Another enzyme, elongase, creates dihomo-gamma-linolenic acid (DGLA). After one more reaction, the end result is PGE1 and 15-hydroxy DGLA, the hormones that reduce inflammation, dilate blood vessels, and inhibit blood clotting. Their strong anti-inflammatory properties help the body recover from injury by reducing pain, swelling, and redness.

Alpha-Linolenic Acid (ALA): The Omega-3 Parent

The body processes alpha-linolenic acid (ALA) in much the same way as it does linoleic acid. However, the D6D enzyme has a higher attraction for ALA than for LA; it will convert ALA 25.

How can we overcome impaired enzymes to prevent hormonal imbalances? Impaired enzymes cannot be fixed, but they can be bypassed by supplementing the diet with the healthful EFAs that don't require the D6D enzyme for processing. For example, a diet high in fatty fish would supply the body with EPA without having to follow the reaction process to receive the beneficial hormones. It would be a direct source of the anti-inflammatory hormones that your body requires.

Omega-3 and Omega-6 Conversion

Linoleic acid (omega-6) and alpha linoleic acid (omega-3) require the D6D enzyme to begin the first step in the reaction (please see the metabolic pathway diagram on page 17), a slow step known as the "rate-limiting step." Without the action of the D6D enzyme, the pathway is blocked and the production of good hormones is altered. There are numerous lifestyle and environmental factors that can impair the D6D enzyme, including the following:

- A high intake of saturated fat and trans-fatty acids
- A high intake of linoleic acid (LA) from refined grocery-store oils, such as corn and soybean oils
- Some pharmaceutical drugs and food additives
- Excess alcohol consumption
- Smoking
- Stress

- Aging (as we grow older, the enzyme becomes less efficient)
- Infant prematurity
- Gender-specific: Recent research shows that testosterone may inhibit the synthesis of long-chain fatty acids; this may explain why learning and behavioral difficulties are greater in boys than girls
- Deficiencies of minerals such as magnesium and zinc, which are crucial desaturase enzyme cofactors
- Conversion of ALA into EPA and DHA is competitively lowered by a high supply of LA

Prostaglandins

DGLA also has the potential to produce arachidonic acid with the help of the delta-5-desaturase enzyme. Prostaglandins are produced within the body's cells by the enzyme cyclooxygenase (COX). There are two COX enzymes, COX-1 and COX-2. Both enzymes produce prostaglandins that promote inflammation, pain, and fever. The prostaglandins and leukotrienes resulting from arachidonic acid work completely opposite from those of DGLA, although they are both part of the omega-6 family. Arachidonic acid produces PGE2 (prostaglandin 2 series), which is proinflammatory, constricts blood vessels, and encourages blood clotting. These properties are important when the body suffers from a wound or an injury because without them you would bleed to death from a cut. Additionally, prostaglandins stimulate nerves that send pain messages to the brain. Many over-the-counter pain relievers, such as aspirin and ibuprofen, are designed to block the production of prostaglandins. However, an excess of the hormones from arachidonic acid can be harmful and may even contribute to disease. The amount of arachidonic acid produced depends on a variety of dietary and lifestyle factors. North Americans tend to consume too much arachidonic acid from red meat, eggs, and shellfish, especially from animals that have not been allowed to graze in green pastures. In fact, we have to worry more about the consumption of arachidonic acid from the plethora of food choices than we do from our body's own enzymatic conversion of LA into arachidonic acid. Individuals who follow a vegetarian diet have more moderate and healthy levels of arachidonic acid and, in turn, fewer proinflammatory prostaglandins.

Leukotrienes

Leukotrienes are another type of inflammatory messenger that direct the white blood cells to the sites of inflammation and do even more damage to the tissue. The more leukotrienes you have, the longer those white blood cells are able to stay alive, doing more damage to the surrounding area. A product of arachidonic acid is LTB4 (leukotriene B4).

In summary, there are many types of inflammatory messengers, but prostaglandins and leukotrienes are the central players in a critical pathway that causes pain and inflammation and can be controlled through the diet. Remember, what you put in your mouth every single day will influence how you feel.

The Inflammation Link

One of the most profound nutrition books I read in the past decade was called *Inflammation Nation* by Dr. Floyd Chilton. He provides a clinically studied eating plan to help rid the body of toxic food that is creating a system of inflammation in the body. The metabolic pathway I described above can also be called the "inflammatory pathway," of which billions of dollars have been spent on research to come out with drugs such as Celebrex and Singulair, as well as aspirin and other nonsteroidal anti-inflammatory drugs (NSAIDs). I found his book fascinating because I am living proof of this epidemic phenomenon of inflammation, which I describe in "My Story" at the end of this chapter.

The Prostaglandin Blockers

As mentioned, there are two types of COX enzymes that turn arachidonic acid into prostaglandins. The first, COX-1, is responsible for a number of the "housekeeping" functions of the body, such as maintaining the thickness of the stomach lining. The other, COX-2, is involved in the production of pain and inflammation. NSAIDs vary in their potency and duration of action, how they are eliminated from the body, how strongly they inhibit COX-1, and their tendency to cause ulcers and promote bleeding. The more an NSAID blocks COX-1, the greater is its tendency to cause ulcers and promote bleeding. Celebrex blocks COX-2 but has little effect on COX-1 and is, therefore, further classified as a COX-2 inhibitor, which causes less bleeding and fewer ulcers than other NSAIDs.

Aspirin is probably one of the best pharmaceutical drugs ever developed; however, it is not without side effects. Unfortunately, aspirin blocks both COX enzymes, which means it prevents COX-1 from doing its maintenance job in the body, even when it stops pain and inflammation, as a result, when you take aspirin your stomach lining suffers. Aspirin is a unique NSAID, not only because of its many uses but also because it is the only NSAID that inhibits the clotting of blood for a prolonged period. This makes it an ideal drug for the prevention of blood clots that cause heart attacks and strokes.

COX-2 drugs such as Vioxx (which has been taken off the market) and Celebrex are not without their side effects either. An eighteen-month study showed that people taking the COX-2 inhibitor Vioxx had an increased risk of heart attack and stroke.[4]

Leukotriene Blockers

As with the prostaglandin blockers, another category of drugs called "leukotriene blockers" came as a result of research into the arachidonic acid pathway. These drugs, known as Singulair and Accolate, prevent leukotrienes from signaling inflammatory cells. However, there are many types of leukotrienes that cause disease, so if you have used these drugs with little success, it could be because they are not blocking the right leukotriene.

Omega-3 Fatty Acid Metabolism

The body processes alpha-linolenic acid in much the same way as it does linoleic acid. Once EPA is produced (please see the diagram on page 17), it can be elongated to DHA. The prostaglandins and resolvins produced from EPA are profound in their anti-inflammatory effects. They are useful as defense mechanisms against trauma and infection. DHA's role is more in the structure and function of the brain and nervous system and is important for infant brain development, prevention of depression, stress reduction, eye function (the retina of the eye has the largest concentration of DHA), and so on.

The New Kid on the Block

Recent studies have shown that additional hormones are produced from AA, EPA, and DHA with potent anti-inflammatory properties outside of prostaglandins and leukotrienes. Lipoxins are derived from AA, resolvins are derived from the omega-3 EPA in response to aspirin, and protectins are derived from DHA; when produced by nerve tissue, protectins are termed "neuroprotectins D1" because they originate from free DHA in the brain.

Resolvins have tremendous practical application for numerous inflammatory diseases, especially rheumatoid arthritis. Research published in 2005 in the *Journal of Experimental Medicine* showed that resolvins inhibit both the migration of inflammatory cells to the sites of inflammation and the turning on of other inflammatory cells.[5] This, however, requires the COX-2 enzyme to function, and if a person is taking a COX-2 inhibitor, it may block the synthesis of resolvins, which would eliminate an important natural anti-inflammatory pathway when your body needs it most. This demonstrates why it is best to let nature take its course and let your body heal itself.

How to Balance Your Omega-6s and Omega-3s

Optimal fat ratios are important to increase the omega-3 and omega-6 content of body tissues. While it is crucial to have all EFAs in our diet, it is important to ensure that we balance the omega-3s and omega-6s.

There is no consensus yet on what the ideal amount or ratio of these essential fatty acids should be in the human diet. However, today we consume a ratio of 20:1 omega-6 to omega-3 fatty acids, which is much different from what it once was. The unbalanced ratio of the modern Western diet promotes numerous chronic diseases such as insulin resistance, obesity, metabolic syndrome, type-2 diabetes, heart disease, and depression because our cells cannot function with the refined, toxic omega-6s found in all processed and convenience foods.

We must try to get back to consuming a ratio of 1:1 up to 4:1 of omega-6s to omega-3s in order to reach our optimum health. In other words, you should be eating up to four times as much of the omega-6s as you do omega-3s. We need to focus on increasing the amount of omega-3s in our diet to offset the overabundance of omega-6s from processed and refined oils. To ensure you are receiving enough omega-3s in your diet, fill your plate with fatty fish. Add nuts, seeds, and seed oils such as flaxseed, hemp seed, and grapeseed oils to your salads, cereals, stir-fries, and sauces.

Hot Nutrition Topic: Does This Mean All Omega-6s Are Bad?

One of the hottest topics in the area of omega nutrition is the misconception that we get too many omega-6s from our diet, and therefore, we don't need to eat as much of them. If you walk away from this book having learned one thing, let it be this: Not all omega-6s are the same. This bears repeating over and over again.

LA, GLA, and AA are all omega-6s, but they each have very different effects and are all found in different quantities in our diet. As mentioned, linoleic acid is plentiful in our diet, and although it is a good fat that has an important job as the parent omega-6, we get enough from our diet, so there is no need for extra supplementation (however, this will be further examined in chapter 4, where I highlight the groundbreaking research on linoleic acid for reducing belly fat).

Eicosanoid Production

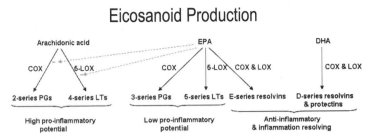

GLA has many important functions for our health. As you will read in my story below, it is a supplement I have used with great benefit, and I want to impress on you that we can't forget about this important omega-6 fat.

My Story

Growing up on a family farm in southern Saskatchewan, Canada, I enjoyed a wonderful, simple childhood with loving parents, a brother and sister, grandparents, food on our table, with our faith as an underlying driver for all we did and believed. When I think back on this time, I have fond memories of the safety and security I felt and how protected I was from the rest of the world.

Our farm, on which my brother toils and labors still today, was and is a source of food supply for the world; canola, flax, wheat, durum, barley, and numerous other amazing crops were and are grown and harvested on our farm, as well as on those of our neighbors. Pesticides, fertilizers, and various other chemicals were used to control pests, weeds, and other natural hazards that threatened to decrease the yield of our precious crops. Little did we know at the time of the long-term effects of and dangers from these chemicals (or if my father did know, maybe he didn't believe it or know that there was an option).

I will never forget the day—I was in seventh grade, it was two weeks after the passing of my grandfather, and my dad was diagnosed with bladder cancer, a diagnosis that would forever change us. I was shocked to learn that my thirty-seven-year-old father had a tumor the size of a grapefruit lodged in his bladder. Stage 3 cancer, possibly stage 4, with a prognosis of six months to live. I had already witnessed my maternal grandmother die from colon cancer, then subsequently my maternal grandfather was diagnosed with bone cancer, then my father's dad died from lung cancer (he was a smoker), and now my own dad. It was frightening because I knew what this meant. How does a twelve-year-old process this information? My parents were strong, and proud, never admitting the long-term consequence of this diagnosis or what this meant for our family. My father battled and battled, and tears still stream down my face when I think of the hair loss, the chemo, the radiation and surgeries, nausea, vomiting, doctors' appointments, exhaustion, and tears that went through my home for five years. My dad was and still is my hero because anyone who can endure the physical pain he dealt with for five years, all while telling his family he is feeling "good," is a hero. In many ways, this was the worst and the best time of my family's life because it changed my dad, his priorities, and what was important. This meant more time together at the dinner table, and more quality, focused time together in general. It also brought us all closer with our faith, and bonded many in our community together. I will never forget the outreach of support and love from all those in Assiniboia, Saskatchewan, especially on March 14, 1995, two days after his passing, when almost 800 people gathered at our local Catholic church to remember my dad. I have always said and always believed that the prairie people are the best.

Now my story begins with my dad and the possible reasons for his early death. Of course we don't know this to be 100 percent true, but many doctors, and groups such as the Environmental

Working Group, cite chemical exposure from pesticides as a leading cause of cancer, not to mention autoimmune disease, cardiovascular disease, and many chronic diseases. The negative health effects are far-reaching, serious, and dangerous.

In my early twenties, I was diagnosed with an autoimmune disease called "mixed connective tissue disease," which presents as a combination of lupus-like symptoms and rheumatoid arthritis symptoms. Pain is the right word to describe how I felt; that, along with fatigue, left me feeling pretty awful and not like a twenty-year-old should feel. The rheumatologist's prescription was a drug called "Plaquenil," and I spent more time visiting specialists in an effort to be proactive and avoid all the negative side effects from the drug, such as lung, kidney, and vision problems, and to be honest, the drug didn't even make me feel better. I was also an avid Advil user; this class of NSAIDs is quite effective in dealing with pain and inflammation, but the side effects range from nausea, vomiting, diarrhea, constipation, dizziness, and headaches to the most serious—kidney failure, liver failure, ulcers, and prolonged bleeding. I still to this day battle with an ulcer that flares up every now and then; however, I am so lucky to have knowledge of natural medicine, and I use a product called "deglycyrrhizinated licorice root extract, (DGL)", which helps to build the mucin layer of the stomach to protect from stomach acid, and it does wonders in healing the ulcer and associated pain.

Nature's Path of Healing

In a way, my autoimmune disease led me down a phenomenal path of healing with nature and food. I started to research natural anti-inflammatory ingredients and came across some amazing research on borage oil, which is rich in GLA, an anti-inflammatory omega-6 fatty acid. This was the first dietary supplement I ever used, and almost fifteen years later, I still use it daily. It has greatly helped manage the pain and inflammation that comes with an autoimmune disease, not to mention numerous other benefits for my skin, hair, nails, and hormones. My journey has also been one of many food and lifestyle changes over the years, from decreasing sugar in my diet and focusing on more fiber and whole foods to increasing protein (I drink two protein shakes per day), and I eat a ton of fish. I believe all of these changes together allow me to be the person of health that I am today.

Food for Thought

- Essential fatty acids are required for optimal functioning of cellular processes, maintaining the integrity and function of the cellular membranes, and producing a balance of hormones that control virtually all body processes.

- The North American diet typically contains too many bad fats (such as those found in red meat, processed foods, and junk food) and contains too little of the good fats found in fresh dark green leafy vegetables, seeds, and nuts.

- The decades of villainizing fat are over. We are now recognizing the importance of healthful fats for preventing and treating many diseases, and this starts with what you eat each day.

Stay Tuned

In chapter 2 we'll take a closer look at fat in our food and how we can get back to eating a full-fat healthful diet, and I will provide solid evidence on the benefits of full-fat dairy products and how to cook with healthful oils.

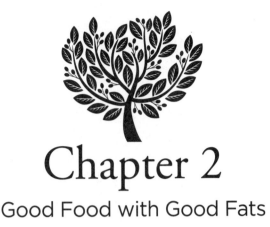

Chapter 2
Good Food with Good Fats

Now that you understand the types of fatty acids and their importance for almost every body function, we can begin to discuss how to incorporate these healthful fats into your diet. Have you ever noticed that your favorite foods are always made better with fats and oils? Without fat in our foods, we wouldn't experience the creaminess of ice cream or the golden crispness of cookies. This is because fat adds qualities to food such as taste, texture, and aroma—all of which make food more palatable and appealing. Fat is an essential part of our diet, so why not enjoy it? Fat also provides a number of beneficial compounds, such as the omega-6 and omega-3 fatty acids, and acts as a "nutrient booster," where it enables the body to absorb fat-soluble nutrients, including vitamins A, E, D, and K, and fat-soluble phytonutrients. Fat-soluble phytonutrients are a group of plant-based compounds that exert potent health benefits. A good example of these compounds is carotenoids, which give dark yellow, orange, and red fruit and vegetables their color. There are over 600 known carotenoids, with the most common being alpha- and beta-carotene, lutein, lycopene, and astaxanthin.

In a perfect world, you will receive all your good fats from your food. Healthful fats are easily consumed from a variety of sources. Dairy, grass-fed meat, avocados, dark green leafy vegetables, fatty fish, nuts and seeds, nut butters, butter, olives, and unrefined expeller-pressed oils are rich in essential fatty acids and can protect you from cancer, diabetes, heart disease, and excess weight.

Essential Fatty Acids and Their Sources

There are plenty of ways to get the good fats that you need to keep you healthy:

Omega-6 Fatty Acids

Linoleic acid (LA): Present in many vegetable oils—safflower (79%), evening primrose (72%), sunflower (65%–75%), corn (57%), hemp (57%), pumpkin (55%), peanut (31%), borage (20%–30%), canola (19%–26%), and olive (8%). LA is abundant in our food supply, so there is no need to supplement. For example, 1 teaspoon (5 mL) of corn oil provides the adult daily requirement of omega-6s; however, most people consume ten to twenty times that amount.

Gamma-Linolenic Acid (GLA): The richest sources of GLA are borage oil (20%–24%) and evening primrose oil (8%–10%). GLA is present in small amounts in human breast milk and some foods, but not high enough that we can maintain our nutritional needs through diet alone.

Arachidonic Acid (AA): Found in high amounts in eggs, fish, and meat. AA is abundant in the food supply, and supplementation is not usually necessary. Too much arachidonic acid can actually be harmful to our health, leading to inflammation and blood clots.

Omega-3 Fatty Acids

Alpha-Linolenic Acid (ALA): ALA is found in flaxseed oil (50%–60%), hemp oil (19%), nuts, dark green leafy vegetables, and wheat germ.

Eicosapentaenoic Acid (EPA) and Docosahexaenoic Acid (DHA): Fatty fish such as salmon, mackerel, sardines, anchovies, halibut, and tuna are common sources. Depending on the fish source, they vary in the amount of EPA and DHA they provide.

Table 1: Food Sources of Saturated and Unsaturated Fats

Saturated	Trans	Monounsaturated
Animal-based foods, including red meat, butter, milk, and cheese. Leaner cuts of meat such as chicken and turkey contain saturated fats, but to a lesser degree. For further clarification on saturated fats, please see chapter 1.	Hydrogenated oils, margarines, and processed and convenience foods such as baked goods, chips, crackers, cookies, and cold cereals. Look for the words "hydrogenated" and "partially hydrogenated" on food labels.	The Mediterranean diet is full of the omega-9 monounsaturated fats. This includes olive oil, avocados, macadamia nut oil, walnuts, almonds, flaxseeds, and hemp seeds.

Polyunsaturated Omega-3s	Polyunsaturated Omega-6s
Free-range meat (contains the omega-3 alpha-linolenic acid), dark green leafy vegetables (romaine lettuce, mixed greens, purslane, spirulina, kale, spinach, Swiss chard, and arugula) soybeans, and nuts and seeds (almonds, walnuts, hemp seeds, and flaxseeds). The longer-chain omega-3s are found in fatty cold-water fish, including salmon, mackerel, and tuna.	Vegetable oils such as canola, corn, safflower, and sunflower oils. Margarines made from these oils, as well as many processed and convenience foods.

Dairy: Low-Fat to Full-Fat

Dairy has become one of the hottest topics in nutrition today. Anyone who has shopped the dairy aisle of the grocery store realizes the plethora of options available for cheese, yogurt, butter, milk, and everything in between. As a young nutrition student, I was taught to reduce consumption of full-fat dairy due to its reputation of contributing to a number of negative health effects, including heart disease and obesity. The negative perception of dairy foods is largely attributed to the high levels of saturated fats found naturally in these products. Saturated fats, until recently, have been linked to an increased risk of cardiovascular disease (CVD). Ultimately, this led to the "low-fat era" of dairy products in which low-fat and fat-free dairy products became an enormous trend—one that shows no sign of slowing. In fact, North Americans currently purchase two and a half times more skim milk, and approximately half as much whole milk as they did in 1975. A growing body of evidence, however, not only reveals that consuming dairy products is good for you, but that it also continues to shine a favorable light on "full-fat" dairy in particular, suggesting that fat is making a comeback where our health is concerned. So what is the "skinny" on full-fat dairy and dairy in general? What are the protective properties in dairy, and how does dairy benefit our health?

Nutrition from the Cow

Dairy products contain a plethora of powerhouse nutrients and beneficial compounds that are important for optimal health. Included are calcium, protein, and numerous vitamins and minerals, such as potassium, phosphorus, magnesium, and zinc, and vitamins A, D, B2, and B12.

In fact, the benefits of consuming the recommended amount of this important food group are largely understated. Recent data obtained from the National Health and Nutrition Examination Survey (2003–2006) found that although calcium can be obtained from nondairy sources such as "calcium-enriched" and "calcium-fortified" foods, the researchers hypothesized that it would be difficult to meet nutritional requirements for a number of additional important nutrients without consuming the recommended intake of dairy products per day. These additional nutrients include protein, potassium, magnesium, phosphorus, riboflavin (vitamin B2), and vitamins A, D, and B12.[1]

Recent US statistics also report that at today's current consumption of dairy products by children aged two years and older, intake of total dairy foods contributes to only about 10 percent of total calories, yet deliver 58 percent of vitamin D, 51 percent of calcium, 28 percent each of vitamin A and phosphorus, 26 percent of vitamin B12, 25 percent of riboflavin, 18 percent of protein, 16 percent each of potassium and zinc, and 13 percent of magnesium.[2] This indisputably makes milk and milk products an economical and nutrient-dense food group.

Research also reveals that a high consumption of dairy products is associated with a reduced risk of several chronic diseases, including heart disease, stroke, diabetes, dementia, and certain forms of cancers (colorectal and bladder). The beneficial effects of dairy consumption are also confirmed by findings from the USDA's 2010 Dietary Guidelines for Americans, which concluded that "moderate evidence shows that intake of milk and milk products is linked to improved bone health, especially in children and adolescents" and "is associated with a reduced risk of cardiovascular disease and type-2 diabetes and with lower blood pressure in adults."[3] A strong positive association has also been observed for dairy consumption and healthy weight management.

Most recently, these beneficial effects were observed in a systematic review and meta-analysis of the published evidence regarding the effect of dairy consumption on weight, body-fat mass, lean mass, and waist circumference (WC) in adults. Sixteen studies were selected for the systematic review and fourteen studies for the meta-analysis. After reviewing the available data, the researchers concluded that the inclusion of dairy products in weight-loss diets had a significant positive effect on weight, body-fat mass, lean mass, and waist circumference in comparison with diets that did not include dairy products.[4]

Emerging evidence also suggests that consuming an adequate intake of dairy products may also be associated with an increased rate of survival.

Calcium King

Of the many nutrients in dairy, the calcium found in dairy deserves special mention. Calcium may be obtained from a variety of nondairy sources. However, calcium found in dairy is one of the most absorbable sources, making it more readily available to the body in comparison with sources such as calcium supplements or fortified foods. Although not fully understood, it is proposed that additional naturally occurring nutrients in dairy, such as vitamin D, magnesium, vitamin B12, potassium, phosphorous, and zinc, may result in a synergistic effect on increasing calcium's absorption and bioavailability. In addition to calcium's well-known beneficial effects on bone health, calcium is also necessary for a number of physiological functions, including blood clotting, transmission of nerve impulses, and regulation of heart rhythms, to name a few.

Aside from the above-mentioned essential nutrients found in dairy, additional bioactive compounds found specifically in the *milk fat* portion of dairy have been shown to favorably affect health. These include conjugated linoleic acid (CLA), trans-palmitoleic acid, butyric acid, and vitamin K2. Thus, the benefits of consuming natural full-fat dairy versus processed low-fat dairy continue to be revealed.

Benefits of Full-Fat versus Low-Fat Dairy

Although low-fat dairy products have been portrayed as a "healthy alternative" to full-fat dairy, researchers have yet to provide concrete evidence that support low-fat dairy products as a heart-healthy food choice that is conducive to weight loss, as portrayed in most media campaigns. On the contrary, during the same time frame that consumption of low-fat dairy skyrocketed, rates of obesity, type-2 diabetes, and heart disease multiplied exponentially. Studies now reveal that the replacement of fat with carbohydrates—as seen with many typical low-fat dairy products (and diets)—actually may negatively affect health.

These negative effects largely stem from the high levels of sugar and low levels of fat present in most processed low-fat foods (including dairy). In the case of low-fat dairy, the removal of fat leaves a higher concentration of milk sugar (lactose). In addition, large amounts of sugar are often added to low-fat dairy products to improve their taste in the absence of the naturally pleasing milk fat. The result is little or no fat to slow the entrance of the lactose and added sugar into the bloodstream, resulting in a large spike in blood sugar levels. When this occurs, the pancreas releases the hormone insulin to transport the sugar in the blood into the body's cells, where it is subsequently used for energy.

When we chronically eat foods high in sugar, the pancreas goes into overtime to produce the insulin necessary to constantly deal with the excess "spikes" in blood sugar. The chronic surge of insulin signals the body that there is plenty of energy available in the form of glucose, and that the body should, therefore, stop burning fat for energy and start storing it—hence the potential for weight gain that is seen more often than not in those who chronically consume high levels of sugar (without fat or fiber to slow its entrance into the bloodstream). Therefore, it is becoming increasingly clear that it may be wise to "ditch" the highly processed low-fat dairy option and take the plunge into the more wholesome natural full-fat dairy choice.

Full-Fat Dairy

From a scientific perspective, the scales now appear to be tipping in favor of consuming naturally produced full-fat dairy. Full-fat dairy has had a long-standing reputation as being "bad for your health" due to its high levels of saturated fats, and the negative effect of saturated fats on the risk of cardiovascular disease.

The belief that saturated fats consumption is associated with an increased risk of CVD is now being viewed as nothing more than a myth. In 2010, the *American Journal of Clinical Nutrition* published a study in which twenty-one studies correlating the risk of heart disease and stroke to saturated fats intake were reviewed. The researchers concluded that "there is no significant evidence for concluding that dietary saturated fat is associated with an increased risk of heart disease or stroke."[5] On the contrary, full-fat dairy intake, despite its high levels of saturated fats, has been associated with favorable effects on metabolic syndrome, diabetes, certain forms of cancer, fertility, and heart disease, to name a few. Following are just a few conditions that studies have demonstrated benefit from consuming full-fat dairy:

Metabolic Syndrome: Metabolic syndrome is a term that describes a combination of at least three of the following five abnormalities that ultimately increase the risk of cardiovascular disease: central obesity, high blood pressure, elevated blood glucose, high triglycerides, and low HDL cholesterol. Cross-sectional data from several studies have strongly suggested that consumption of whole milk, and particularly yogurt, is associated with a lower incidence of metabolic syndrome.

Cardiovascular Disease and Stroke: In a recent study investigating the effects of dairy consumption and patterns of mortality in Australian adults, the investigators found that participants who had the highest intake of full-fat dairy had a lower rate of death from cardiovascular disease when compared with participants having the lowest intake of full-fat dairy.[6] A recent study published in the *American Journal of Clinical Nutrition* found that individuals with the highest levels of milk fat intake were at lower risk of developing a first heart attack. For women, the risk was reduced by 26 percent, while a 9 percent reduction in risk was seen for men.[7] In previous studies by these same researchers, consumption of full-fat dairy was also associated with a reduced risk of stroke, particularly in women.

Diabetes: An intriguing study recently investigated the association of serum levels of trans-palmitoleic acid (trans-palmitoleate), a type of fat most commonly found in full-fat dairy, and incidence of diabetes in 3,630 participants of the Cardiovascular Health Study. The researchers observed that participants who consumed the highest amount of whole-fat dairy had the highest levels of circulating trans-palmitoleic acid in their blood. High circulating levels of trans-palmitoleic acid were associated with lower adiposity, higher HDL cholesterol levels, lower triglyceride levels, lower C-reactive protein levels, lower insulin resistance, and an overall lower incidence of developing type-2 diabetes.[8]

Fertility: Researchers have observed that consuming full-fat dairy products may also positively affect fertility in women. A recent prospective study followed 18,555 married premenopausal women for an eight-year period. After dietary assessment via food-frequency questionnaires, women who consumed high intakes of high-fat dairy had a significantly lower incidence of anovulatory (no ovulation) infertility in comparison with women who consumed low intakes of high-fat dairy.[9]

The numerous beneficial effects of full-fat dairy can be attributed in part to a number of bioactive compounds found specifically in dairy fat. Included are the following:

Conjugated Linoleic Acid (CLA): The richest sources of CLA are meat and dairy products derived from animals that are grass fed. CLA is found primarily in the fat fraction of these products, and, therefore, levels of CLA are lacking in their low-fat dairy counterparts. Of the twenty-eight CLA isomers that have been identified, the two most commonly studied for their positive health effects are the cis-9, trans-11, and the trans-10, cis-9 isomers. The beneficial effects of CLA on a number of conditions and chronic diseases, including various forms of cancer, cardiovascular disease, blood lipid profiles, osteoporosis, insulin resistance, inflammation, and body weight (and composition), have been well established.

Trans-Palmitoleic Acid: Trans-palmitoleic acid is a type of fatty acid also found in the fat of dairy (milk, cheese, butter) and meat. Exciting new research continues to reveal its favorable effect on lowering the risk of developing type-2 diabetes. Again, full-fat dairy and meat provide the highest levels of this important fatty acid.

Vitamin K2: Vitamin K2 (menaquinone) is a fat-soluble vitamin found in high levels in fermented foods, such as natto (fermented soybeans), and fermented dairy, such as blue and feta cheeses and hard cheeses that have been aged (including Cheddar). Additional sources of K2 include eggs, as well as chicken and beef (particularly the livers of these animals). Research is continuing to reveal the beneficial effects of vitamin K2 on bone health, cardiovascular disease, brain function, and cancer prevention, to name a few.

Butyric Acid: Butyric acid (aka butyrate) is a short-chain fatty acid that is produced by our intestinal bacteria in response to dietary fiber. Although I haven't discussed probiotics in this book, healthy bacteria create a healthy gastrointestinal tract, which is essential for overall health. In terms of dietary sources, butyric acid is found in high quantities in natural butter. Butyric acid has consistently shown to protect against colorectal cancer, and to favorably affect hypercholesterolemia, insulin resistance, and ischemic heart disease.

Dairy Alternatives

Even though I am a proponent of dairy, not all individuals can tolerate dairy. For example, my son Matteo has a dairy allergy, not just a lactose sensitivity but a full-blown allergy to the protein. He breaks out in a red rash on the face and bum and becomes very congested. For many individuals, the casein and whey molecules are too large and very difficult to digest. Hence, cow's milk is one of the top ten allergens.

Therefore, dairy alternatives represent a growing market in North America, with new options being introduced regularly. If you cannot tolerate dairy due to allergies or intolerances—or simply do not like the taste of dairy—a few great dairy alternatives are listed below. Keep in mind that none of the following are significant sources of protein (except soy milk, which I don't recommend), and most are fortified to provide vitamins, minerals, and calcium. Also keep in mind that many contain added sugars in the form of rice syrup, evaporated cane juice, or other natural sugars, so read your labels and choose the unsweetened option if possible.

Almond Milk: Almonds are rich in a number of important nutrients, including magnesium, potassium, manganese, copper, vitamin E, and selenium. With this in mind, almond milk may be one of the more nutritious dairy alternatives on the market. With regards to taste, almond milk has a pleasing, light, nutty flavor.

Rice Milk: Rice milk is one of the "pioneers" of dairy alternatives and is often recommended for individuals prone to allergies. This is because rice is one of the most hypoallergenic foods around. This is opposed to soy milk and almond milk, which may trigger reactions in individuals with allergies to soy and nuts.

Hemp Milk: Hemp milk is one of the "new kids on the block" as a dairy alternative. It has also developed quite a following due to its texture and taste. Furthermore, hemp milk has an impressive nutritional profile and contains small amounts of both omega-3 and omega-6 fats. Just remember to give the carton a good shake before drinking as the fats tend to separate from the milk.

Soy Milk: Soy milk has a full, slightly nutty flavor; however, I don't advocate the consumption of soy unless it is non-GMO fermented soy. Try to consume soy products such as miso, tempeh, and fermented soybeans, and avoid all soy milk, soy cheese, soy meat, soy chips, soy crackers, soy ice cream, and all the other nonfermented forms of soy. The fermentation process is essential in aiding the body to break down soy. Too much nonfermented soy may contribute to hormonal imbalance due to the soy isoflavone's phytoestrogenic properties. Unfortunately, the scope of this topic is far too large to expand further; however, if you are unsure, you may want to do a bit more digging on the health dangers of nonfermented soy.

Coconut Milk: Coconut milk is one of the newest dairy alternatives to hit the market and has a fresh, creamy, "exotic" taste. Expect this dairy option to develop a large fan base.

Goat's Milk: Goat's milk is sweet in flavor with a slight salty undertone. Goat's milk is rich in calcium, protein, and numerous vitamins and minerals. For reasons not entirely understood, people who cannot tolerate cow's milk often have no problem tolerating goat's milk. Goat's milk may, therefore, be a suitable dairy alternative for many individuals.

Greek Yogurt

Greek yogurt has become very popular with its rich, creamy texture that leaves us feeling as though we just indulged in a decadent treat. Greek yogurts are produced the same way as traditional cow's milk yogurt, with one extra step in which the yogurt sits in cheesecloth bags to allow the whey protein to be filtered out of the yogurt, resulting in a thick consistency much like sour cream.

One of the biggest nutritional assets of Greek yogurt is its high-protein content, offering up twice as much as regular yogurt. This alone makes it an excellent snack for children, whose diets are typically low in protein. Yogurt is also an excellent source of calcium, with some brands providing up to 50 percent of the daily calcium recommendation. Active probiotic cultures are found in many yogurts, such as Greek yogurt, and offer multiple health benefits for the digestive and immune systems.

Greek yogurt can be used as a dip for fruit; in other dips, such as tzatziki; mixed into smoothies; or as a replacement for sour cream in recipes.

The yogurt aisle can be one of the most daunting in the store, with numerous choices, multiple flavor options, low-fat, no-fat, high-fat, artificially sweetened, natural, organic, goat's, cow's, soy, and now Greek yogurt options. My first choice is the Greek variety because, in my opinion, it is nutritionally superior on many levels, not to mention more satisfying because of the creamy texture and absolutely delicious taste. Keep in mind when buying Greek yogurt that the flavored versions usually contain more sugar, so you can opt for the plain kind and flavor it yourself with added fruit, such as berries, and honey or agave nectar.

Traditionally, Greek yogurt is higher in milk fat, at least 10 percent, but in North America we tend to prefer it from either zero to 2 percent fat. I tend to side with the Greeks on this one and enjoy my dairy and yogurt in their full-fat varieties, which I also believe to be better for our children than the low-fat options.

Butter versus Margarine: Your Mom Knows Best

The age-old debate as to whether butter is better than margarine continues to wage on in consumers' minds, leaving most of us perplexed by one more nutrition puzzle we can't find the missing piece for.

Let's set the record straight once and for all. Butter is better than margarine. Regardless if you are trying out the "trans fat–free, reduced-saturated, and reduced-cholesterol" margarines that overwhelm the "dairy" aisle of the stores, you still can't go wrong with good ol' fashion butter.

Butter contains many healthful components, including lecithin, which aids the body to break down cholesterol. It is also a rich source of vitamin A, which is necessary for the healthy functioning of the adrenal and thyroid glands.

If you look at the fat component of butter, you will see that it is made from cream and contains a wide range of short- and medium-chain fatty acids, as well as monounsaturated and some polyunsaturated fatty acids. The dangers of butter's saturated fats components have been blown out of proportion, but keep in mind that not all saturated fats are created equally.

Vegetarian Sources of Omega-3s

When we think of omega-3 fats, the obvious sources that come to mind are fish and flaxseed. Less obvious, however, are the wide variety of dark green leafy vegetables that are also rich in these important fats. In addition to their omega-3 content, leafy greens are a powerhouse of nutrients, containing a plethora of vitamins, minerals, and important phytonutrients that aren't typically found in traditional omega-3 sources. Phytonutrients are plant-based compounds—usually the pigments that give fruit and vegetables their vibrant color—that exert potent antioxidant and anti-inflammatory effects. These powerful compounds have consistently been associated with a reduced risk of numerous chronic diseases. Dark green leafy vegetables that are gaining popularity as alternate sources for omega-3 fats include arugula, kale, purslane, seabuckthorn, spinach, spirulina, and Swiss chard.

Arugula

Also known as "salad" or "garden rocket," arugula is a dark green leafy vegetable of Mediterranean origin. Arugula also belongs to the genus *Brassica*, alongside other popular vegetables, including kale, cauliflower, broccoli, and cabbage. Young, tender arugula leaves feature a sweet, nutty flavor; whereas mature arugula leaves have a stronger, more peppery spicy flavor. Fresh arugula is available in the markets year round. Look for crisp green young leaves, and avoid mature leaves as they tend to be tough and bitter. Arugula is popular in salads and sandwiches; added to soups, stews, and pastas; and steamed as a side vegetable. I usually buy mixed green blends that contain arugula, or I love to use arugula with fennel and freshly cut strawberries. Arugula is another leafy green that is rich in omega-3 fats. In addition, arugula is rich in vitamins A, C, K, and folate, as well as the minerals calcium, iron, potassium, magnesium, and manganese. Arugula is also a powerhouse of phytonutrients such as indoles, thiocyanates, sulphorane, and isothiocyanates. Together, these potent compounds have demonstrated favorable effects on the prevention of hormone-dependant cancers, including cancers of the prostate, breast, cervix, ovaries, and colon. Following are some of the key nutrients found in arugula:

Per 100 grams fresh (approximately 1 serving):

Omega-3 fatty acids (total): 170.0 mg
Vitamin A: 2,373 IU
Vitamin C: 15.0 mg
Vitamin K: 109.0 mcg
Folate: 97.0 mcg
Calcium: 160.0 mg
Iron: 1.5 mg
Potassium: 369.0 mg
Magnesium: 47.0 mg
Manganese: 0.3 mg

Kale

Kale has become all the rage with health-food enthusiasts. It is a dark green leafy vegetable of the genus *Brassica*, which also encompasses broccoli, Brussels sprouts, cauliflower, and cabbage. Prior to the Middle Ages, kale was one of the most commonly consumed vegetables in all of Europe. Kale is often eaten raw (alone or in salads), and it can also be cooked. I love eating kale that has been turned into "chips" by drizzling with olive oil and sea salt and then baking in the oven for a couple minutes. Nutritional yeast also tastes fantastic sprinkled over kale.

Availability of kale is highest during winter months (November to March) because exposure to cooler temperatures enhances both its flavor and quality. As for its nutritional profile, kale stands out as a rich source of omega-3 fats. Kale is also abundant in vitamins A, C, K, and B6 and the minerals calcium, potassium, copper, and manganese. Kale also possesses many phytonutrients that have proven health benefits. Included are the carotenoids lutein and zeaxanthin, as well as sulforaphane—a phytonutrient with potent anticancer properties. Following is an overview of important key nutrients found in kale:

Per 100 grams fresh (approximately 1 serving):

Omega-3 fatty acids (total): 180.0 mg
Vitamin A: 15,376 IU
Vitamin C: 120.0 mg
Vitamin K: 817.0 mcg
Vitamin B6: 0.3 mg
Calcium: 135.0 mg
Potassium: 447.0 mg
Copper: 0.3 mg
Manganese: 0.8 mg

Purslane

Purslane is a dark green leafy vegetable with oval leaves and a flavor often described as slightly tart and lemony. Purslane is indigenous to India, but it currently grows freely over much of the globe. Because purslane grows well in poor-quality soil, it is often considered a weed in many regions of the world. Peak availability of purslane is during warm summer months; however, there are also winter varieties available. Purslane is popular as a raw ingredient in salads, and it is particularly popular in Mediterranean cuisine. Research has revealed that this leafy green "packs a punch" where nutrients are concerned. In fact, purslane possesses exceptionally high levels of the omega-3 fatty acid alpha-linolenic acid (ALA). In addition, purslane contains the omega-3 fatty acid EPA (eicosapentaenoic acid). EPA is mainly found in fish and some algae; however, purslane has been found to contain exceptionally high levels of this important fatty acid (0.01 mg/g) for a leafy vegetable. Purslane is also rich in vitamins A and C and the minerals calcium, magnesium, potassium, manganese, and iron. In terms of phytonutrients, purslane is abundant in beta-cyanins and beta-xanthins—both of which act as potent antioxidants that have been shown to exert anticancer properties. Following is an overview of select key nutrients found in purslane:

Per 100 grams fresh (approximately 1 serving)

Omega-3 fatty acids (total): 300.0–400.0 mg
Vitamin A: 1,320 IU
Vitamin C: 21.0 mg
Calcium: 65.0 mg
Magnesium: 68.0 mg
Potassium: 494.0 mg
Manganese: 0.3 mg
Iron: 2.0 mg

Seabuckthorn

Seabuckthorn has gained popularity in recent years as the new kid on the block, providing "omega-7s." Seabuckthorn is indigenous to the Himalayan region, where it has been cherished for centuries by native Tibetans. Known as the "holy fruit of the Himalayas," this plant has been touted for its remarkable nutritional profile. The nutritional properties of seabuckthorn are primarily found in the berries, leaves, and seeds of the plant. Collectively, the seabuckthorn plant contains over 190 biologically active compounds, including vitamins, minerals, potent phytochemicals, and omega-3 fats. Each part of the seabuckthorn plant contains varying levels of omega-3 fatty acids. The berries, which appear as bright orange-red clusters on the branch, produce fruit oil that consists of approximately 2 percent omega-3 as alpha-linolenic acid (ALA). The seed oil consists of approximately 32 percent ALA, and the leaves consist of approximately 19 percent ALA. Of the 190 active compounds, there are also generous levels of beta-carotene (provitamin A); vitamins B1, B2, C, D, and K; and omega-3, -6, -7, and -9. Seabuckthorn also contains a large variety of carotenoids, flavanoids, phenols, terpenes, and a minimum of twenty mineral cofactors. The favorable health effects of seabuckthorn have been well documented, particularly in areas such as cardiovascular health, immunity, anticancer properties, memory, anti-inflammatory properties, and skin health.

Spinach

I make sure that in my family we eat organic spinach every day. It is such a nutrition powerhouse that I love adding it to our fruit and veggie smoothies, in what I call the "ultimate energy elixir." Spinach is believed to have originated in ancient Persia, and its presence can be traced back as early as AD 647. This popular leafy vegetable has tender, crisp, dark green leaves and is a favorite ingredient among chefs around the world. Spinach is most available during winter months, and is commonly used raw or cooked in a wide array of dishes. The nutritional value of spinach is highly rated, including a rich profile of phytonutrients. The impressive nutrient profile is highest when spinach is fresh, steamed, or quickly boiled. As with other select leafy greens, spinach is rich in omega-3 fatty acids. Spinach also contains high levels of vitamins A, C, E, K, B2, and folate, as well as the minerals iron, calcium, potassium, magnesium, and manganese. Spinach also contains an impressive profile of potent phytonutrients, such as alpha-lipoic acid, polyphenols, lutein, zeaxanthin, glutathione, coenzyme Q10, and chlorophyll. Following is an overview of important key nutrients found in spinach:

Per 100 grams fresh (approximately 1 serving):

Omega-3 fatty acids (total): 138.0 mg

Vitamin A: 9,376 IU

Vitamin C: 28.1 mg

Vitamin E (alpha-tocopherol): 2.0 mg

Vitamin K: 483.0 mcg

Vitamin B2: 0.2 mg

Folate: 194.0 mcg

Iron: 2.7 mg

Calcium: 99.0 mg

Potassium: 558.0 mg

Magnesium: 79.0 mg

Manganese: 0.9 mg

Spirulina

One of the world's oldest foods, spirulina, is a microalgae that typically grows naturally in alkaline water. Although spirulina can be consumed as a whole food, it is currently popular as a dietary supplement and is often consumed in either pill (capsule or tablet) or powdered form. I usually add powdered spirulina to my spinach energy elixir. It is amazing at detoxifying, providing energy, and healing the adrenal glands. Spirulina is a concentrated superfood and possesses a remarkable nutritional profile. Aside from being a concentrated source of omega-3 fats and a valuable source of protein, spirulina is also high in vitamins B1 and B2 and minerals iron and copper. Spirulina is also loaded with powerful phytonutrients, such as beta-carotene, chlorophyll, zeaxanthin, and phycocyanin. It is important to note that a little goes a long way with regards to this wonder food. Daily dosages for dried spirulina vary anywhere from a teaspoon (or less) to a tablespoon. Following is an overview of important key nutrients in spirulina:

Per 7 grams dried (approximately 1 tablespoon):

Omega-3 fatty acids (total): 57.6 mg

Protein: 4.0 g

Vitamin B1: 0.2 mg

Vitamin B2: 0.3 mg

Iron: 2.0 mg

Copper: 0.4 mg

Swiss Chard

Swiss chard is a succulent dark green leafy vegetable of

European origin. Also known as "spinach chard" or "silverbeet," this leafy green belongs to the beet family, which also includes table beets, sugar beets, and garden beets. The peak season for Swiss chard availability is June through November. Chard can be harvested at various stages of maturity. The more mature large leaves are generally tougher and suitable for sautéing and cooking, whereas the young tender leaves are great for use in salads. Compared with many other leafy greens, Swiss chard is only a moderate source of omega-3 fatty acids. However, what Swiss chard lacks in omega-3 fats, it makes up for in its powerful nutrient profile. Swiss chard is rich in vitamins A, C, and K and minerals such as iron, potassium, magnesium, and manganese. Chard also provides a multitude of potent phytonutrients, including alpha- and beta-carotene, lutein, and zeaxanthin. Following is an overview of important key nutrients in Swiss chard:

Per 100 grams fresh (approximately 1 serving):

Omega-3 fatty acids (total): 7.0 mg

Vitamin A: 6,116 IU

Vitamin C: 30.0 mg

Vitamin K: 830.0 mcg

Iron: 1.8 mg

Potassium: 379.0 mg

Magnesium: 81.0 mg

Manganese: 0.4 mg

Ways to Increase Good Fats in Your Diet

- Eat cold-water fatty fish, such as wild salmon, tuna, mackerel, sardines, or anchovies two times per week.

The American Heart Association recommends this to prevent heart disease. If you don't like the taste of fish, try a toxin-free fish oil supplement. Aim for 1 gram of omega-3s per day. The American Heart Association recommends up to 3 grams of omega-3s per day to lower triglycerides.

- Consume a GLA supplement; for example, borage oil, to ensure levels of the anti-inflammatory omega-6s.

- Flaxseeds are the best source of omega-3s in the plant kingdom.

- Eat nuts such as walnuts, Brazil nuts, butternuts, and macadamia nuts.

- The more green the better. The dark green leafy vegetables are good sources of omega-3s. Try romaine lettuce, mixed greens, seabuckthorn, spirulina, purslane, kale, Swiss chard, and arugula.

- Make your own salad dressing using flaxseed oil.

- Avoid refined grocery-store oils. These oils are heavily processed and contain an abundance of unhealthful omega-6s, which can lead to insulin resistance. Use coconut oil and grapeseed oil as your primary high-heat cooking oils, and extra virgin olive oil for low-heat cooking and garnishing.

- Try to get in the habit of cooking and steaming veggies and then adding healthful oils such as organic flaxseed oil and extra virgin olive oil as a garnish. This enhances the flavor, texture, and appeal of the vegetables.

- Make "better butter" by combining flaxseed oil or other EFA-rich oils with your butter. Use as a spread. (Please see page 10 in chapter 1 for the recipe.)

- When possible, consume free-range meat, which

contains higher levels of omega-3s than grain-fed meat. The grain fed to the animals produces meat that is rich in proinflammatory omega-6s, which change the fatty acid profile of the meat and lead to the imbalance of fats.

Natural saturated-fats sources, such as coconut oil and butter, have vital and protective properties. While it is important to limit excess consumption of saturated fats, especially long-chain ones found in red meat (they clog arteries), a balanced diet should contain the beneficial saturated fats such as those found in butter.

If you are concerned about the cholesterol in your butter, be aware that 80 percent of our cholesterol is made in our liver, whereas only 20 percent is from our food. In fact, long-chain saturated fat and trans fats increase our cholesterol more than dietary cholesterol.

What You Have Learned in This Chapter

- We should embrace full-fat and look for opportunities to incorporate healthful fats into our diet.

- Bring dairy back into your diet—the full-fat kind. Enjoy Greek yogurt as a delicious snack.

- Omega-3s and omega-6s are found in a variety of foods, such as nuts, seeds, dark green leafy vegetables, cold-water fatty fish, and healthful oils. Each time you eat a meal or snack, try to incorporate healthful fats.

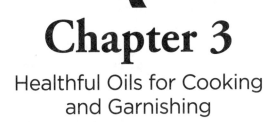

Chapter 3
Healthful Oils for Cooking and Garnishing

The A to Z of Cooking with Fats and Oils

One of the most important considerations is how to use healthful oils to maximize their goodness. Despite the multitude of oils currently on the market, unfortunately, a one-size-fits-all policy does not apply to any one cooking oil. When you can, buy organic, expeller-pressed, unrefined oils and store them properly (I cover the storage of oils in more detail at the end of this chapter). Fats and oils have different properties, such as smoke point, taste, and fatty-acid profile, making each individual fat and oil suitable for different cooking applications.

Smoke Point

The smoke point of a fat or oil is the temperature at which the oil will begin to break down, producing a bluish smoke. Heating oils changes the structure of the fat molecules, making them toxic and unusable by the body; at this point, the oil becomes harmful to consume and should be discarded. It is important to use the right oil under the right conditions. The more refined an oils is, the higher the smoke point becomes. Fats and oils with a higher smoke point can, therefore, endure higher heat during the cooking process. When cooking with fats and oils, it is, therefore, important to pair the right cooking oil with the right cooking application. For instance, certain oils are not heat-stable and are, therefore, more suitable in no-heat applications, such as spreads, dips, dressings, and marinades. Following are several cooking oils, their beneficial properties, and the application to which they are best suited.

Almond Oil

Almond oil has a very subtle roasted-almond flavor and aroma and is commonly used in traditional oriental cooking. Almond oil is also a rich source of monounsaturated fatty acids (MUFAs) and vitamin E.

Smoke Point: 420°F / 216°C

Best Applications: Most suitable for medium- to high-heat cooking, such as sautéing and frying.

Avocado Oil

Avocado oil possesses a soft, nutty flavor and vibrant green color. The fatty-acid profile of avocado oil is very similar to that of olive oil, being rich in heart-healthy MUFAs that lower both bad (LDL) and total cholesterol levels. In addition, MUFAs may help normalize blood clotting, insulin levels, and blood sugar levels.

Smoke Point: 510°–520°F / 266°–271°C

Best Applications: Due to its exceptionally high smoke point, avocado oil is one of the best oils for high-heat applications, such as sautéing and frying. Avocado oil is also great in dressings and dips.

Camelina Oil

I am so thankful to the always-inspiring Janet Jacks of Goodness Me Market in Ontario for giving me a heads-up on what I would call the breakthrough oil of the cooking and functional-food industry. Camelina oil is extracted from *Camelina sativa* seeds, which contain greater than 50 percent polyunsaturated fatty acids (PUFAs), of which 35 to 40 percent is the omega-3 alpha-linolenic acid (ALA).[1] It originated in parts of northern Europe and central Asia. It is a nongenetically modified organism (non-GMO) oilseed that is now also grown in my home province of Saskatchewan. In contrast with all the other food and cooking oils I describe, camelina oil contains high levels of ALA and has a favorable ratio of omega-3 to omega-6 as it contains about 15 percent of the omega-6 LA. In addition to having an excellent balance of beneficial fatty acids, camelina oil contains high levels of tocopherols (vitamin E), which confer good oxidative stability. Scientists in 1995 showed that camelina and sunflower contained 17.40 and 13.29 mg per 100 g seed, respectively, with the notable difference that camelina had a high content of beta-tocotrienol/gamma-tocopherol (14.28 mg/100 g seed), whereas sunflower was higher in alpha-tocopherol (12.89 mg/100 g seed).[2,3,4,5]

In the past, we thought that levels of ALA were the most critical factor in determining an oil's stability during frying, but we now know that the other side to the story is the content and composition of minor components such as tocopherols, sterols, and pigments. Camelina oil is an important functional-food ingredient, providing beneficial omega-3 fatty acids without the instability problems associated with other plant omega-3 sources, such as flaxseed oil, and fish oils.

From a health-benefit perspective, camelina oil increased the proportion of ALA, EPA, and DHA in fatty acids of blood lipids and also reduced LDL cholesterol in people with mild to moderately high cholesterol levels, as well as reduced their triglyceride levels.[6,7,8]

There is demand in the functional food market for omega-3 oils; however, the oxidative deterioration (rate of rancidity) of the omega-3s, which results in undesirable flavors, the development of degradation products such as polymers and cyclic fatty acids, and the loss of nutritional benefits. Therefore, incorporating an oil such as camelina into a range of cooking applications becomes very important from a quality and health-benefit perspective.

Smoke Point: 475°F / 246°C (it has a shelf life of 12 to 15 months without refrigeration)

Best Applications: Camelina oil carries a light, earthy fragrance and tastes slightly nutty on the palate. Other words used to describe the taste are "fresh," "green," "asparagus-like," "hint of cauliflower," and "incredibly unique." Camelina is a culinary oil. It can be used for cold applications, such as spreads, dips, marinades, and dressings. It can also be used at moderate- to high-heat levels because of its high smoke point. However, in deep-frying applications, "fishy notes" were observed.

Canola Oil

Canola is derived from the seed of the canola plant and is a very mild-flavored, light golden-colored oil. Canola oil is also rich in omega-6, omega-3, and MUFAs.

Smoke Point: 400°F / 204°C

Best Applications: Canola oil is great as an all-purpose cooking oil, where it can be used in many applications. Canola oil can be used for "all-temperature" cooking (low to high heat), as well as in salads, dips, and sauces.

Chia Seed Oil

Chia seed oil is derived from the seed of the chia plant and is a dark golden color. Chia seed oil is a rich source of omega-3 fatty acids (59%), particularly alpha-linolenic acid (ALA). In fact, chia seed oil is the richest plant source of omega-3s.

Smoke Point: 338°F / 170°C

Best Application: Chia seed oil is not suitable for frying or other cooking; it is, therefore, best used in no-heat applications, such as in dressings and dips, or as a dietary supplement.

Coconut Oil

Coconut oil is a heavy oil that is colorless when heated (white at room temperature) with a slight hint of coconut flavor. Despite its high levels of saturated fats, the health benefits of this wonder oil have been well established. Coconut oil has been shown to exert beneficial effects on heart health, increase metabolism and weight loss, and boost your immune system, to name a few.

Smoke Point: 350°F / 177°C

Best Applications: Coconut oil can be used for medium-high-heat cooking and is especially great when used to cook pancakes, sauté veggies, and cook fish, especially halibut and shrimp. Coconut oil is also used in baking and as a "better butter" spread on toast and muffins (please see page 10 in chapter 1 for the recipe). It's also great on popcorn!

The Truth about Coconut Oil

Coconut oil has quickly become one of my favorite fats, which is why I feel it deserves a bit more attention in this chapter. I started applying it liberally to my "baby bump" when I was pregnant with my first son. It is such a soothing and moisturizing fat, and I believe it helped to nourish and protect my skin from stretch marks. I especially love the coconut-based body care line Fiji Organics. This was also the time when I started to incorporate coconut oil into my cooking, and my kids know that when the coconut oil comes out first thing in the morning, they are getting homemade whole-wheat waffles. Coconut oil is also delicious to use when cooking halibut or other white fish, prawns/seafood, and stir-fried Asian veggies, and as a topping for popcorn. My new cookbook, *The Full-Fat Solution Recipe Book*, uses coconut oil in many of the recipes.

In many parts of the world, the coconut tree and its products have for centuries been an integral part of life, and it has come to be called the "Tree of Life." However, in the last few decades, the relationship between coconut fats and health has been the subject of much debate and misinformation. Unfortunately, coconut oil has been wrongly branded as a nutritional evil for many years. As previously mentioned, it is a medium-chain fat that is easily digested and used by the body. In short, whereas other fats are stored in the body's cells, the medium-chain fats in coconut oil are sent directly to the liver, where they are immediately converted into energy. So, when you eat coconut oil, your body uses it immediately to make energy rather than store it as body fat. Because this quick-

and-easy absorption puts less strain on the pancreas, liver, and digestive system, coconut oil heats up the metabolic system. Dr. Joseph Mercola suggests that since coconut oil actually speeds up metabolism, your body will burn more calories in a day—this will contribute to weight loss, and you'll have more energy.

Experts in the field of fat and nutrition show that virgin coconut oil is rich in lauric acid, a proven antiviral, antibacterial, and antifungal agent that is very beneficial in attacking viruses, bacteria, and other pathogens and builds the body's immune system.

In the 1960s, data collected from research was misinterpreted, concluding that coconut oil raised blood cholesterol levels. In fact, it was the omission of essential fatty acids in the diet that caused the observed health problems, not the inclusion of the coconut oil. More recently, subject groups studied in the South Pacific for their regular use of coconut oil in the diet exhibited low incidences of coronary artery disease and low serum cholesterol levels.[9] A study in *Asia Pacific Journal of Clinical Nutrition* in 2011 reviewed the beneficial lipid effects in 1,839 premenopausal women in the Philippines. The researchers found that dietary coconut oil intake was positively associated with high-density lipoprotein (HDL) cholesterol, especially among premenopausal women, suggesting that coconut oil intake is associated with beneficial lipid profiles. It was *not* significantly associated with low-density lipoprotein (LDL) cholesterol or triglyceride values.[10] Little or no change is evident in cholesterol levels when an EFA-rich diet contains nonhydrogenated saturated fats. Coconut oil is naturally saturated, so it does not need to go through hydrogenation.

Flaxseed Oil

Flaxseed oil is a medium-dark golden color with a delicious nutty flavor. It is nature's richest source of plant-based omega-3 fatty acids.

Smoke Point: 225°F / 107°C

Best Applications: Flaxseed oil is not suitable for use in heat applications as the heat will denature the healthful fats. It is, therefore, recommended as a supplement, or added to smoothies, yogurt, salad dressings, dips, and sauces, and used as a garnishing oil.

Ghee (Clarified Butter)

Ghee, or clarified butter, also known as "drawn butter," is the pure liquid golden-colored butterfat that is derived from unsalted butter. Ghee is produced by melting unsalted butter over low heat until the butter breaks down into three layers. The top frothy layer is the whey proteins, which are skimmed off and discarded. The milk solids sink to the bottom to form a milky sediment. The remaining middle layer is the pure golden-colored butterfat known as "ghee" or "clarified butter."

Smoke Point: 375°–485°F / 191°–252°C (depending on purity)

Best Applications: Clarified butter is great for high-heat cooking, in baking, and in creamy sauces such as hollandaise.

Grapeseed Oil

Grapeseed oil is derived from the seeds of grapes, often during the wine-making process. This healthful oil has a clean, light, fruity flavor and is rich in phytosterols. Phytosterols are plant-based compounds that have potent beneficial effects on heart health.

Smoke Point: 392°F / 200°C

Best Applications: Grapeseed oil is a medium- to high-heat cooking oil that is also excellent in salad dressings. Use this oil in dressings when you don't want the flavor of the oil to be too overpowering.

Hazelnut Oil

This light-brown oil generally has a slightly sweet, nutty (hazelnut) taste and is very popular in French cooking. Hazelnut oil is high in MUFAs and is also considered a specialty oil, being more expensive than the average cooking oil.

Smoke Point: 430°F / 221°C

Best Applications: Hazelnut oil, despite its high smoke point, is best used in no-heat applications such as salad dressings, dips, and baked goods. Due to its strong flavor, it can be mixed with other light-flavored oils, such as canola oil, to mellow or lighten its flavor.

Hemp Seed Oil

Hemp seed oil is derived from the seed of the hemp plant and is dark to light green in color, depending on how refined the oil is. Hemp seed oil contains a wonderful balance of the essential omega-6 and omega-3 fatty acids—linoleic acid (LA) and alpha-linolenic acid (ALA). In addition, it possesses two additional fatty acids that are beneficial for health—gamma-linoleic acid (GLA) and stearidonic acid (SA).

Smoke Point: 338°F / 170°C

Best Applications: Hemp seed oil is not suitable for cooking/ frying and, therefore, should be reserved for use in no-heat applications, such as dressings and dips.

Olive Oil

Olive oil is a staple of the Mediterranean diet and one of the oldest culinary oils. Olive oil differs greatly in quality, flavor, color, and aroma, depending on the extent of refining (e.g., extra virgin, virgin, light, extra light). Olive oil is also rich in "heart-healthy" MUFAs and, like grapeseed oil, contains varying levels of phytosterols that benefit our health (less refined olive oil has higher levels of phytosterols).

Smoke Point: 329°–464°F / 165°–240°C (depending on level of refinement; more refined oil will have a higher smoke point)

Best Applications: Although olive oil has a relatively high smoke point, the flavor starts to break down at high temperatures. The use of this oil should, therefore, be reserved for low- to medium-heat cooking, as well as no-heat applications, such as dressings, sauces (e.g., pesto), and dips. Olive oil is also great drizzled over pasta and as a dip for fresh bread.

Palm Oil

There are two types of palm oil—palm oil (also known as palm fruit oil) and palm kernel oil. Palm oil is derived from the African palm fruit, is red-orange in color, and has a strong, unique flavor. Palm oil is commonly used in the cuisine of the Caribbean, Central and South America, and West Africa. Palm kernel oil, on the other hand, is extracted from the kernel of the palm and is light yellow in color with a mild flavor. Both oils are high in saturated fats; however, like coconut oil, the saturated fats in these oils are considered heart healthy because they do not negatively affect cholesterol levels.

Smoke Point: 446°F / 230°C

Best Applications: Both varieties of palm oil possess a high smoke point and, therefore, can be used for all-temperature applications. Due to their unique flavor (particularly palm fruit oil), palm oil can also be used as a flavoring ingredient in certain dishes.

Peanut Oil

Peanut oil is derived from pressed cooked peanuts and is very light yellow in color, with a very subtle scent and flavor. Peanut oil is also high in both MUFAs and PUFAs and is primarily used in Asian cooking.

Smoke Point: 450°F / 232°C

Best Applications: Peanut oil is great in all high-heat cooking applications (sautéing, frying) as well as in dressings and dips.

Pistachio Oil

Pistachio oil is emerald green in color and has a nutty aroma and strong, full flavor. Pistachio oil is rich in MUFAs and vitamin E and also contains small amounts of omega-3s. Pistachio oil is more of a specialty item as it is higher priced and less available than your average cooking oil.

Smoke Point: 338°F / 170°C

Best Applications: Pistachio oil is not suited for heat applications, but it is suitable for all no-heat applications. Pistachio oil pairs nicely with salads containing citrus and/or fresh goat cheese, as well as grilled fish and shellfish. Pistachio oil is also commonly used in many Middle Eastern dishes.

Pumpkin Seed Oil

Pumpkin seed oil is derived from roasted, hulled, pumpkin seeds and is dark green/orange-red in color with a rich, nutty flavor. Pumpkin seed oil is rich in both omega-3 and omega-6 fats and is often consumed as a dietary supplement, particularly by men due to its favorable effects on prostate health. Pumpkin seed oil is also rich in the potent antioxidant zeaxanthin, which is often used along with lutein for eye health.

Smoke Point: 266°F / 130°C

Best Applications: Pumpkin seed oil is not generally used for heat applications as heat will destroy the flavor of the oil. Use instead in dressings, dips, or drizzled over dishes as a "final touch" to add a distinctive flavor.

Rice Bran Oil

Rice bran oil is derived from the germ and inner husk of the rice plant. Rice bran oil is medium to light yellow and has a pleasant nutty flavor. Rice bran oil is high in MUFAs, PUFAs, and vitamin E. In addition, this oil is high in an antioxidant known as gamma-oryzanol that has been shown to favorably affect cholesterol levels, triglyceride levels, and insulin resistance.

Smoke Point: 490°F / 254°C

Best Applications: Rice bran oil has an exceptionally high smoke point and is, therefore, suitable for all types of cooking applications, including frying, sautéing, and baking. This healthful oil is also suitable in all no-heat applications, such as in dips and dressings and used as a dipping oil.

Safflower Oil

There are two varieties of safflower oil. Both are derived from the seed of the safflower plant and are light golden in color with a neutral flavor. The first variety of safflower oil is higher in PUFAs (oleic acid). These two oils are suitable for different applications, so it is important to know which type of safflower oil you are purchasing. The label on the bottle will indicate the amount of oleic acid compared with the amount of linoleic acid.

Smoke Point: 450°F / 232°C

Best Applications: High-oleic safflower oil is a great oil to use for all heat applications, and it can also be used in most no-heat applications, such as dressings and dips. High-linoleic safflower oil is not suitable for heat applications, is best used in dressings and dips, and is commonly used to make margarines and mayonnaises.

Sesame Oil

There are two varieties of sesame oil—light sesame oil derived from untoasted sesame seed, and dark sesame oil derived from toasted sesame seeds. Light sesame oil has a light, nutty flavor and is often used in Middle Eastern dishes. Dark sesame oil has a fuller flavor and is often used in traditional Asian cuisine. Both varieties are high in PUFAs.

Smoke Point: 450°F / 232°C

Best Applications: Light sesame oil is suitable for all heat applications, as well as in dressings and dips. Dark sesame oil, however, is not suitable for heat applications and is used primarily in small amounts to add a unique flavor to food.

Sunflower Oil

Sunflower oil is derived from pressed sunflower seeds and is light yellow in color and virtually odorless and tasteless. Sunflower oil is rich in PUFAs and vitamin E and is a good all-purpose cooking oil.

Smoke Point: 450°F / 232°C

Best Applications: Sunflower oil is a suitable oil for all heat applications, as well as all no-heat applications, such as dressings and dips.

Tea Seed Oil

Tea seed oil, also known as "camellia oil" or "tsubaki oil," is pale amber-green in color with a sweet, herbal aroma. Tea seed oil is rich in MUFAs, vitamin E, and antioxidants and is the primary cooking oil in the southern provinces of China and many regions of Japan.

Smoke Point: 485°F / 252°C

Best Applications: With its high smoke point, tea seed oil is great for high-heat applications such as frying and sautéing. In addition, it is also suitable for use in dips, dressings, and marinades.

Walnut Oil

Walnut oil is medium–dark yellow in color with a rich, nutty flavor. Walnut oil is rich in MUFAs, antioxidants, and heart-healthy omega-3 fats.

Smoke Point: 400°F / 204°C

Best Applications: Walnut oil is not suitable for use in heat applications as the flavor will break down when heated. Walnut oil can, therefore, be used in many no-heat applications, such as dressings, marinades, and dips, and to add flavor to desserts.

Table 2: How to Use Good Oils
(*My favorite choices in each category)

No Heat	Low Heat 215°F / 102°C	Medium Heat 325°F / 163°C	High Heat 375°F / 191°C
Condiments/Salad dressings	Sauces/Baking	Light sautéing or add after cooking	High-heat frying
*Flaxseed	Sunflower	Almond	*Tea seed
Hazelnut	*Olive	*Coconut	Ghee
Pistachio		*Grapeseed	Palm
Hemp seed		Light sesame	High-oleic safflower oil
Walnut		Canola	Avocado
Pumpkin seed		Butter	Rice bran
Chia seed		*Camelina	Sunflower
			Peanut

To minimize the damage caused by heat, cook with as little oil as possible and never take the oil beyond its smoke point because doing so will destroy its healing properties. Ideally, oils should be added after cooking, and after the pot has been removed from the heat. The addition of these oils will give your food the satisfying flavor and texture that we crave. Begin by incorporating nut and seed oils into your recipes and use appropriate oils for cooking.

How to Store Good Oils

Healthful oils are essential to our health, but they are more temperamental than the inferior oils you see on the supermarket shelves. Light, air, and heat can destroy them. Nature packages these oils in seeds, and left intact, these oils will sometimes keep for years without spoiling.

When we extract the oil from such seeds, we need to make sure the oil is shielded from the destructive elements before pressing and until the oil is opened. Special care needs to be taken in processing, packaging, and storing oils rich in essential fats to prevent the oil from turning rancid. Rancid oil has a scratchy, bitter, fishy, or paint-like taste, and may be accompanied by a characteristic unpleasant smell. When oil has turned rancid, dozens of by-products form, with toxic or unknown effects on our bodies' functions. In fact, rancid oils, if consumed, have been associated with negative health effects such as arterial damage, inflammation, certain forms of cancer, and premature aging. It is, therefore, imperative that cooking oils are properly stored to minimize exposure to these negative factors. Below are general guidelines to maximize shelf life and overall quality of your cooking fats and oils:

- Choose fresh EFA-rich oils that have been pressed and packaged in the dark, in the absence of oxygen, and with minimal heat, and packaged in opaque bottles.
- At home, once you have opened a bottle of good oil, it should be stored in the refrigerator to protect it from

turning rancid. Refrigerated oils will generally turn cloudy when cold; however, simply remove the oil an hour or two prior to use and it will return to its original liquid state. If refrigeration is not possible, store all oils in a cool-cold, dry, dark place (not a warm pantry!).

- Prior to opening, the oil is safe in a bottle on a shelf at room temperature; this is because during the packaging process, the oil was packaged in the absence of the destructive elements and then sealed tightly.

- Be sure to keep your healthful oils away from the stove, and do not leave them on top of the fridge or microwave.

- With regards to butter, store unused portions in the freezer as butter will maintain its quality only for approximately two weeks in the refrigerator.

- Keep in mind that darker-colored oils will go rancid more quickly than lighter-colored oils.

- Unrefined oils will generally keep for three to six months once opened if properly stored in a cool, dark location.

- Refined oils will keep twice as long as unrefined oils— generally six to twelve months once opened when stored in a cool, dark location.

- Oils high in polyunsaturated fats have a shorter shelf life than oils high in monounsaturated or saturated fats.

- Unopened cooking oils generally have a shelf life of one year if properly stored in a cool, dark, dry place.

There are many quality brands in both Canada and the United States that have been pressed and packaged using these exacting procedures. (Please see the resources section on page 193.)

What You Have Learned in This Chapter

- Not all oils are created equally. When selecting an oil, consider the application and smoke point.

- Coconut oil is an excellent option for cooking and body care.

- How to store good oils to keep them fresh and preserve their quality.

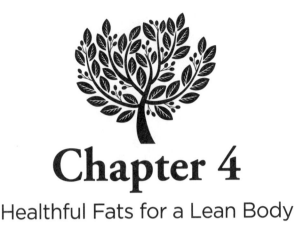

Chapter 4

Healthful Fats for a Lean Body

The Skinny on Fad Diets

Atkins, Beverly Hills, Cabbage Soup, Cider Vinegar, Eat Right 4 Your Type, Grapefruit, Ornish, South Beach, Sugar Busters, Zone, and the list goes on and on. I'm sure most of you have heard of these diets, and some of you may have tried them. We are obsessed with our weight. We spend more than US$100 million annually to find our magic weight-loss bullet. We spend more effort, time, and money than ever before, yet we continue to grow in size. Poor nutrition, specifically related to dietary fat, bears most of the responsibility for the surge in overweight individuals. The latest and greatest diet crazes promoting high protein low protein, high carbohydrate/low carbohydrate, herbs, stimulant products, cleanses, and tonics are emotionally and physically destructive, and more often than not, they simply don't work. In many cases, once you go off the diet, not only do you regain the weight lost but you add some extra as well. The diet industry's success is built on our failures.

But why didn't these fad diets help you lose weight or keep the weight off? Fad diets are generally so unrealistic and so unpleasant they cannot be maintained for the long term. Most of us trying a fad diet will stop eating the diet because it's too restrictive in food choices, boring, expensive, and overall a stressful experience. A recent study published in the *Annals of Internal Medicine* showed there is little evidence to support the use of many commercial weight-loss programs.[1] Studies show that one-third to two-thirds of weight lost is usually regained within one year, and almost all weight is regained within five years. Diets are considered a success only if weight loss is maintained without damaging your overall health. Your food program should satisfy all your nutritional needs, meet individual taste and habits, minimize hunger, and boost energy. The cornerstone to successful weight loss is enjoying your lifestyle—every day, by enlisting in a program and lifestyle change that you feel you can maintain for the long haul. If you feel that what you are doing today cannot be maintained for the next six months to one year, then it likely is not the right program for you. Eat healthfully; move your body, yet still get plenty of rest; drink water throughout the day; take your supplements; have a positive attitude of gratefulness; and rely on your faith. When you combine all of the above, your body will respond with a healthy weight and optimal health.

Our Growing Waistlines

Obesity is considered to be the most common nutritional disorder in the industrialized world today. According to the World Health Organization, for the first time ever the number of overweight individuals exceeds the number of malnourished.[2] According to the National Institutes of Health, more than 60 percent of Americans are overweight,[3] and, unfortunately, these deadly statistics don't show any signs of slowing down. This epidemic is a time bomb for future explosions in cardiovascular disease, which is the number one killer in North America, and type-2 diabetes. Remember, North Americans are the most overfed, undernourished people in the world.

Taking Stock

To discover more about your food and activity habits, answer the following questions:

1. Do you eat fish and lean meat, such as poultry, at least three times a week?
   ___ No ___ Yes

2. Do you eat breakfast every day?
   ___ No ___ Yes

3. Do you eat whole grains instead of white or refined grains?
   ___ No ___ Yes

4. Do you incorporate fish-oil supplements into your dietary regimen?
   ___ No ___ Yes

5. Do you avoid all fried foods as much as possible?
   ___ No ___ Yes

6. Do you eat three to five meals per day?
   ___ No ___ Yes

7. Do you eat fast food less than once a week?
   ___ No ___ Yes

8. Do you pay attention to portion sizes?
   ___ No ___ Yes

9. Do you follow a healthful eating plan and avoid going on and off diets?
   ___ No ___ Yes

10. Do you set aside at least thirty minutes, three times a week for physical activity?
    ___ No ___ Yes

Your Score:

Count up the number of checks you have in column 2 (yes). What was your score? ____

What does your score mean?

8 to 10 checks: Fantastic! Keep up the good work.

5 to 7 checks: You're on the right track, but its time to start considering some changes.

0 to 4 checks: Uh-oh. Take time now to make some changes.

Fat Cells Are the Key

The human body contains about 30 billion fat cells. We all have the same number of fat cells, but the difference between individuals is how much fat is stored inside those cells. Our fat cells have an unlimited ability to keep growing and expanding. In order to stop the uncontrolled growth of our fat cells, we need to ensure we are eating the right types of food, moving our bodies every day, and improving our metabolism with a body built out of healthful fats that will create a healthy cell structure.

Nutrition researchers are extremely frustrated with the "eat fat, get fat" mantra. This ignores the science that has proven bad fats are bad for your health and good fats are good for your health. Remember, not all fats are created equally. Healthful, long-chain fats from omega-3s and certain omega-6s can promote the use of stored fat for energy, rev up your metabolism, secrete satiety hormones, and shrink your fat cells.

Fat Metabolism

When we consume fat, the gastrointestinal tract breaks the fats in the triglyceride form down into free fatty acids by enzymes known as lipases. The fatty acids are absorbed by the intestinal cells, where the lymphatic system and the liver produce fatty complexes to transport these fatty acids throughout the body. The fatty acids derived from high arachidonic acid and trans fats are the main sources of fat storage in the body. Conversely, when our diet contains higher amounts of beneficial fats found in healthful oils, it discourages fat storage and encourages fat burning. Research has shown that varying the omega-3s' and omega-6s' availability to the body can be responsible for, and influence weight loss associated with, increasing the amount of healthful fat in the diet through (1) lipogensis (breakdown of fat in the body), (2) insulin sensitivity, (3) adipocyte differentiation (fat cell number and size), (4) the neuroendocrine system, and (5) the balance between energy intake and energy expenditure.

Trans Fats and Obesity

Trans fats promote obesity and insulin resistance because our bodies can't recognize them since they are shaped differently from natural fats, such as unsaturated fats. Trans fats crowd out the essential fats from the cells. Polyunsaturated fats determine the fluidity of the cells. When there are fewer essential fats, the cells become rigid and hard, thereby reducing the number and sensitivity of insulin receptors. When insulin receptors become less sensitive to insulin, blood glucose levels remain high, leading to type-2 diabetes. Trans fats increase the size of fat cells, and large fat cells have fewer insulin receptors and store more fat than normal fat cells.

If you want to prevent obesity and the very serious complications associated with it, you should substantially reduce your intake of trans fats. Typical foods containing trans fats include packaged and convenience foods, such as chips, crackers, cookies, commercial baked goods, and fast food.

Arachidonic Acid and Obesity

The dietary status of many overweight people is such that the eicosanoid (hormone) pathways are driven toward the production of proinflammatory hormones (if you need a refresher, reread chapter 1). This may occur as a consequence of dietary deficiency of certain polyunsaturated fats, or as a consequence of alterations in the ratio of omega-6s and omega-3s. Studies show that essential fatty acids can affect the release of insulin. The insulin-releasing effect of fats decreases with the degree of unsaturation, meaning the more saturated a fat is, the less chance the pancreas has of releasing insulin, which is why the polyunsaturated fats do a better job of enabling insulin secretion.

Numerous theories have been suggested for the relationship between fats and insulin resistance, including changes in membrane fluidity (i.e., the polyunsaturated fats make the cells more fluid compared with saturated and trans fats, which create rigid, hard cells), the number of insulin receptor sites, and the increased activity of insulin receptors (i.e., polyunsaturated fats make the insulin receptor sites more active). Research has shown that as the omega-6 to omega-3 ratio decreases, insulin resistance improves.

Omega-3s and Belly-Fat Loss

Research has found omega-3s to be powerful weight-loss agents, helping overweight individuals shed unwanted pounds. In both Inuit and Japanese populations, their intake of EPA and DHA were high and the incidence of obesity and its related diseases low. One twelve-week intervention trial studied the effects of omega-3s from fish oil in combination with aerobic exercise three times a week. Study participants were overweight and had metabolic syndrome. The results showed that the total proportion of fat in the body, particularly in the abdominal region, was reduced significantly in the fish-oil-plus-exercise group, but not by fish oil alone or exercise alone. The researchers concluded that omega-3s in fish oil can switch on enzymes specifically involved in oxidizing or burning fat, but they need a driver (exercise) to increase the metabolic rate to lower body fat.[4]

Omega-3s: Increase Your Body's Satiety Hormones

Appetite control is one of the most important factors involved in the success of nutrition strategies for obesity. Omega-3 fatty acids have been reported to modulate appetite. They are major components in the transport of appetite-regulating molecules, such as dopamine, which are related to receptor affinity. Omega-3s can interact with neuroendocrine factors that are involved in something called the "brain-intestinal loop signals" related to energy metabolism such as insulin, ghrelin (the hormone that makes you feel hungry), or leptin (the hormone that signals satiety). In a study published in the journal *Appetite*, participants who ate a dinner rich in omega-3s felt less hungry and more full directly after, and still two hours later, than the participants who were fed a dinner with low omega-3s.[5] (Think dark green leafy vegetables, nuts and seeds, and fatty fish such as salmon or halibut as the ideal diet to help maintain satiety). This study indicates that omega-3s (mainly EPA and DHA) can modulate hunger hormones.

Researchers have confirmed multiple ways in which omega-3s help with weight loss:

- Fish oil omega-3s stimulate secretion of leptin, a hormone that decreases appetite and promotes the burning of fat.

- Fish oil omega-3s enable burning of dietary fats by helping the body move fatty acids into body cells for burning as fuel.

- Fish oil omega-3s encourage the body to store dietary carbohydrates in the form of glycogen, rather than as hard-to-lose body fat.

- Fish oil omega-3s reduce inflammation, which is known to promote weight gain.

- Fish oil omega-3s enhance blood sugar control by increasing the insulin-producing cells' sensitivity to sugar.

- Fish oil omega-3s flip off genetic switches that promote inflammation and storage of food as body fat.

- Fish oil omega-3s help the body transport glucose from blood to cells by increasing the fluidity of the cell membranes.

- Fish oil omega-3s exhibit anti-obesity effects.

In summary, the researchers concluded that omega-3s are one of the best dietary weight-control aids discovered to date.

Omega-6s: Why GLA Aids in Weight Loss

As mentioned in chapter 1, GLA is an omega-6 fatty acid found primarily in borage and evening primrose oils. Numerous research studies have examined the role of GLA for improving health, specifically in the area of weight loss. In the 1980s there were many early reports published in several medical journals, such as the prestigious *New England Journal of Medicine*,[6] that focused on GLA as a natural aid to weight reduction. Scientists such as Dr. David Horrobin, a former professor of medicine at the University of Montreal, and Dr. M. Afzal Mir, a researcher and consultant at the Welsh National School of Medicine in Cardiff, identified two calorie-burning mechanisms that GLA helps to regulate. Simply put, the first involves a metabolically active fat known as brown adipose tissue (or BAT), which is underactive in overweight people. GLA can activate BAT to burn calories. The second is the ATPase metabolic process, commonly referred to as the "sodium pump," which GLA also stimulates for more calorie burning. Amazingly, the sodium pump can use up nearly 50 percent of the body's total calories. Dr. Horrobin believes that nearly one-third of all overweight people are metabolically impaired, interfering with the burning of excess calories.[7]

Studies have demonstrated that GLA from borage oil causes less body fat to accumulate. In one GLA study, individuals lost from 9.6 to 11.4 pounds (4.4 to 5.2 kg) over a six-week period.[8] GLA is a safe, nonstimulating way to stimulate the body's metabolic activity and burn fat.

These studies show that obesity is linked to low GLA levels, and supplementation can correct or normalize these levels. Furthermore, supplementation in obese animals reduces food intake and weight gain.[9] A researcher from Japan in a study published in the *Journal of Nutrition* confirmed that dietary GLA could reduce body fat by increasing the metabolism of BAT and that GLA may affect enzymes involved in the metabolism of fat, as well as the metabolism of glucose.[10] Perhaps most interesting of all is the hypothesis that GLA, like other fatty acids, has the potential to elevate levels of serotonin, a brain chemical that contributes to the feeling of fullness. By elevating serotonin, you will feel satiated sooner, eat less, and not be tempted to overindulge.

GLA Keeps the Weight Off

A study published in the *Journal of Nutrition* assessed whether GLA supplementation would suppress weight regain following weight loss in obese individuals. As we know, keeping the weight off is often difficult, depending on the way in which weight was lost in the first place. Fifty formerly obese humans were placed in two different groups and given either 890 mg/d of GLA (5 g/day borage oil) or 5 g/day of olive oil (control group) for one year. It was found that GLA from borage oil did help to keep the formerly obese individuals' weight gain off.[11]

As we know, GLA produces anti-inflammatory effects, which may have been instrumental in weight gain suppression, especially in view of recent studies that suggest an association between obesity and markers of inflammation. Elevated levels of C-reactive protein (CRP) (blood measure of inflammation) and white blood cells have been observed in obese adults when compared with normal-weight people. People with a high body fat mass, a large waist, and high visceral fat, as well as high levels of fat in their fat cells, experience low-grade chronic inflammation. When people lose weight, typically CRP and white blood cells decrease. GLA has also been shown to decrease CRP and white blood cell levels.

High Linoleic Acid Safflower Oil Beats Belly Fat

In chapter 1, I discussed the controversy that exists with omega-6s and how they have been wrongly branded as a nutrition evil. The important thing to remember is that not all fats are created equally, and neither are all omega-6s. While we want to decrease our consumption of refined, toxic-overloaded omega-6 oils, along with foods that are high in arachidonic acid (they promote inflammation), research has been quite favorable on the benefits of GLA (from borage and evening primrose oils). Recent research also highlights the belly-fat-fighting effects of high linoleic acid found in safflower oil.

Safflower oil yields nature's richest source of linoleic acid (yes, it is also used to produce the isomers in conjugated linoleic acid [CLA] discussed in this chapter). A study published in the *American Journal of Clinical Nutrition* in 2009 involving thirty-five women who were postmenopausal, obese, and type-2 diabetics (yet none were using insulin to control their diabetes) compared the effects of two oils, high linoleic acid safflower oil (different from the high oleic version of safflower oil that is more commonly available as a cooking oil), and CLA (known for stimulating lipolysis, or the breakdown of fats in various parts of the body, especially the hips, thighs, and buttocks region, yet has not been overly effective at reducing fat in the belly region.)

The researchers gave 8 grams of either oil to each group for sixteen weeks, with a four-week washout period, followed by crossing the group over to each receive the other oil. The women were instructed to not change their diet or exercise to be able to accurately assess the benefits of the oils.

The results were very positive and a little surprising as the equivalent of two teaspoons (10 mL) of oil rich in linoleic acid had a significant benefit on the women's body composition. The women lost between 2 and 4 pounds (0.9 and 1.8 kg) of belly fat, simply by taking the high linoleic safflower oil, which translates into an approximate 6.35-pound (2.9 kg) loss of trunk adipose (also known as belly fat). Safflower oil also increased lean tissue (muscle) by an average of about 1.4 pounds (0.6 kg).[12] Practically speaking, this means the women using the safflower oil not only lost belly fat but also gained lean muscle mass. (Remember, the more muscle, the more calories are burned at rest, which is a good thing.)

Linoleic Acid Increases Important Belly-Fat Hormones

Adiponectin is gaining popularity in the nutrition research world as an important belly-fat hormone that can modulate a number of important metabolic processes, including blood sugar regulation and the breakdown of fat, especially belly fat. Overweight individuals, those with type-2 diabetes, and the aging population tend to have lower levels of adiponectin because it naturally decreases as we age. The study examining the effects of safflower oil found, it also improves adiponectin levels by an incredible 23 percent. This may be a very plausible explanation for the reduction of belly fat.

Our goal is to nutritionally support adiponectin levels because this important belly-fat-fighting hormone also has anti-inflammatory effects on the cells lining the walls of the blood vessels. High blood levels of adiponectin are associated with a reduced risk of heart attack. We know that systemic inflammation triggers fat storage; therefore, an essential component of any diet needs to focus on reducing body inflammation.

Adiponectin may also improve the number of mitochondria, our bodies' energy-producing factories within muscle cells, thereby improving metabolism.

Spot-Reducing Belly Fat with Safflower Oil

Up until now, the idea of spot-reducing belly fat, and fat in other areas of the body, has been ignored by most nutrition and exercise experts. The groundbreaking research described above may open up an entirely new theory since safflower oil was proven to blast belly fat.

There are many mechanisms worth examining, but I believe, based on what we know about the ability of healthful fats to build healthy cells, the supplementation with safflower oil improved the cell membrane function and triggered the body to burn fat. When cell membranes become stiff because of the consumption of unhealthful fats, cells lose their ability to hold nutrients, electrolytes, and even water. The lack of fluidity in the membranes also impairs their ability to communicate with other cells and affects how they are influenced by hormones such as insulin. For example, hormones and communicating molecules that increase the ability of the cells to burn energy or fat may be impeded; the end result is a slowdown of metabolism and an accumulation of fat within the cells. The increase in fluidity allows more movement of insulin receptor sites on cell membranes and, therefore, an improvement in the ability of insulin to bind to them. This increase in affinity is a possible contributing factor to the effects of safflower oil. Improving cell membrane fluidity can bring cell membranes back to healthy functioning. This can be done by changes in diet and supplementing with healthful fats such as linoleic safflower oil.

The study noted that it took thirty days before detectable levels of linoleic acid were found in the blood, after which time cell membranes can be properly formed from these healthful fats. Don't expect to see results from omega-3 and omega-6 supplementation for at least one month. Once the cell membrane structure starts to be built by healthful fats, the results will be profound. In the case of this study on safflower oil, maximum results were achieved between the twelve- and sixteen-week marks.

Safflower Oil Improves Blood Sugar Control

Linoleic acid enhances blood sugar control by increasing the insulin-producing cells' sensitivity to sugar. As this study demonstrated, a drop in fasting blood sugar levels in the participants using safflower oil was significant and could impart enormous benefits for the prediabetic population. Interesting new research being done in the biotechnology sector may shed more light on the possible mechanisms of action of this plant. SemBioSys Genetics is currently using a type of safflower oil to produce human insulin. Human insulin derived from safflower oil is currently going through Phase I and II trials on human test subjects. Developing an efficient low-cost substitute for safflower oil could significantly change treatment options for people all over the world. Within the safflower family of molecules there are structures similar to human insulin. This is possibly one of the mechanisms in which safflower oil lowers fasting blood sugar, and helps to mobilize stored belly fat.

Coconut the Weight Off

As I mentioned in chapter 3, coconut oil has become one of my favorite fats. It is beneficial for skin health and great for cooking, and now research shows that when this healthful fat is incorporated into your diet, benefits for your waistline are achievable.

In a study published in the journal *Lipids* in 2009, women with abdominal obesity were given 30 mL (2 tbsp) of coconut oil or soybean oil over a twelve-week period. They were also instructed to decrease calories and walk for fifty minutes per day. The group using the coconut oil showed a reduction in their waist circumference as well as a higher level of HDL (good cholesterol) and a lower LDL:HDL ratio. The researchers concluded that supplementing with coconut oil does not cause dyslipidemia (altered blood fat levels) and seems to promote a reduction in abdominal obesity.[13]

It is important to remember when incorporating coconut oil as a supplement that it *must* replace another fat in the diet. For example, if you were using canola oil as your main source of cooking fat, then the coconut oil would be an excellent replacement option.

Another study on coconut oil investigated its efficacy in weight reduction and its safety of use in twenty obese but healthy Malay volunteers. After four weeks of virgin coconut oil use, their waist circumferences were significantly reduced with an average decrease of 2.86 cm (1.13 in.).

Conjugated Linoleic Acid (CLA) for a Lean Body

As mentioned in chapter 2, conjugated linoleic acid (the term for linoleic acid isomers, in which two of the double bonds are conjugated) is an important omega-6 fat that occurs naturally in full-fat dairy foods and grass-fed beef and lamb; it is produced by the intestinal bacteria of these animals when they convert omega-6 linoleic acid into CLA. Humans cannot convert linoleic acid into CLA, so we must rely on the foods we eat or dietary supplements of CLA. Unfortunately, the CLA content of dairy and meat products has declined over the last few decades due to increases in antibiotic use in animals and changes in their food supply from grass to grain, which decreases CLA levels by 80 percent.[14] In addition, throughout the past twenty years, many misguided by the low-fat diet mantra avoided the only dietary sources of CLA available: meat and dairy products such as whole milk, butter, and cheese.

CLA is available today as a dietary supplement, made by converting the high linoleic acid content of either sunflower or safflower oils into CLA (commercially available CLA contains a mixture of cis-9, trans-11 and trans-10, and cis-12 CLA, and approximately 40 percent of each of the two isomers). To date, there are over 500 published research studies supporting CLA's ability to exert positive effects on fat loss, prevent and control type-2 diabetes, protect against heart disease, reduce the risk of atherosclerosis, and modulate the immune response. It may also inhibit the growth of certain kinds of cancers, such as breast, prostate, and colon.

CLA is thought to break down fat inside the fat cells (known as lipolysis) and redistribute it. CLA is particularly beneficial for fat in the hips, thighs, and butt region, especially in women. One study found the reduction of the equivalent to eight packs of butter lost in the hip and thigh region when using CLA.[15] The key is consistent use and patience because it does not work overnight. As well, generally speaking, at least 3 grams (0.1 oz.) of CLA isomers per day are needed.

CLA Stops Weight from Coming Back

Unfortunately, with many diets and supplements, regaining the weight, and even more than was initially lost, is a big problem with significant health risks. How can we lose the fat and keep it off without having to maintain strict diets and excessive amounts of exercise? In a study on eighty overweight people, participants who were using CLA regained the weight in a statistically significant ratio of 50 percent muscle to 50 percent fat. Those who were not given CLA gained more of their weight, at 75 percent fat and only 25 percent lean muscle.[16] Remember, muscle weighs more than fat but is more metabolically active. The more lean muscle on the body, the more calories will be burned at rest.

Eat Dairy, Lose Weight

I discussed the concept of incorporating full-fat dairy in chapter 2, and in summary, I do recommend dairy consumption for those trying to lose weight. More and more research is suggesting the more dairy food consumed, the less likely your chances of being overweight. Although the researchers cannot explain what is responsible for this association, they say that calcium in the dairy products may have some role to play.

Researchers from the Shahid Beheshti University of Medical Sciences in Tehran assessed dairy consumption and features of metabolic syndrome in a study of 827 men and women. People consuming the most dairy were more than a third less likely to have a large waist size, and almost 30 percent less likely to have high blood pressure. A growing body of research suggests that eating dairy foods may prevent weight gain. They found that the incidence of metabolic syndrome was 29 percent less likely among people with the highest dairy intake.[17]

However, many people are lactose intolerant—that is, they lack the enzyme lastase necessary to digest the lactose (milk sugar), or they are allergic to the milk protein casein. If you are lactose intolerant, make sure you are receiving the necessary calcium from a supplement.

Food recommendations for achieving a lean body:

Vegetables (5 to 7 servings): Choose green foods more often. Start lunch and dinner with a green salad. Tomatoes and cucumbers are considered free vegetables, so you can eat as many of these as you like.

Protein (5 to 6 servings, or each time you eat): Grass-fed and free-range beef and lamb; free-range chicken, turkey, and eggs; wild fish; beans or lentils; and whey protein. Eat protein at each meal to balance blood sugar levels. Protein and fiber should be consumed together.

Healthful Fats (4 to 5 servings): Nuts and seeds; avocados; fatty fish; oils such as flaxseed oil, extra virgin olive oil, macadamia nut oil, and coconut oil; and butter. Many healthful fats are also good sources of protein. Focus on the unsaturated fats such as the omega-3s and omega-9s. Supplement with an omega-6 borage or evening primrose oil supplement to get the good omega-6s that are missing in the diet. Avoid using soy and corn oils because they contain too much of the omega-6s linoleic acid and arachidonic acid, which fuel inflammation.

Whole Grains (3 to 5 servings): Fibrous choices only. Increase fiber consumption to 25 to 30 grams (about 1 ounce) per day. Limit your carbohydrate consumption to what you can actually burn, because what you don't burn will be stored as fat.

Dairy (2 to 4 servings): Choose full-fat organic dairy foods more often. Try incorporating Greek yogurt, cottage cheese, and kefir into your diet. They are even better than milk because of their beneficial bacteria. In recent studies, dairy food consumption has been linked to lowered risk of metabolic syndrome. If you can't tolerate dairy, ensure you are taking a calcium supplement to replace the calcium you aren't receiving in your diet.

Fruit (2 to 3 servings): Choose berries and other fibrous fruit. Fruit plays a much less significant role because of its sugar content. Of the two servings, you should consume at least one serving of berries. Avocados are an exception as they are the only fruit that contains the healthful monounsaturated fats, along with vitamins and minerals. So although avocados are considered a fruit, they can also be used as part of your healthful fat serving.

Other Recommendations:

1. Consume a diet rich in whole, raw foods that have gone through minimal processing. They provide a greater variety of nutrients and bring our diet back to how our ancestors used to eat.

2. Reduce daily calorie consumption by 500 calories to safely lose 1 pound (0.5 kg) per week. Combine fewer calories with burning an additional 500 calories per day during exercise, and you can lose 2 pounds (1 kg) per week. If you weigh more than 175 pounds (79 kg), it is safe to lose more than 2 pounds (1 kg) per week.

3. Eat five to six small meals per day. If you are in the initial phases of weight loss, you may want to consider replacing one or two meals per day with a whey protein shake.

4. Avoid starchy or sugary foods—get rid of everything white in your cupboards.

5. Avoid hydrogenated oils (trans fats) and junk foods (high-calorie, low-nutrient foods). Junk foods and processed foods are sent directly to your bloodstream and cause a rapid increase in blood sugar levels and insulin production.

6. Use whey protein powders to help stabilize blood sugar levels.

7. Eliminate artificial sweeteners; switch to natural sweeteners such as stevia, xylitol, and agave nectar.

8. Limit salt intake.

9. Limit alcohol consumption.

10. Exercise daily—try to burn 250 to 500 calories per day. Combine aerobic, strength, and stretching exercises.

11. Drink lots of water—eight glasses per day

12. Supplement with probiotics, a multivitamin, and omega-3s from fish oil every day. These are your foundational nutrients.

13. Get plenty of sleep. Scientific studies increasingly link lack of sleep to the obesity epidemic.

What You Have Learned in This Chapter

- For years, we thought that removing fat from the diet would be the golden ticket for losing fat on the body. However, we now know that we need healthful fat in order to lose body fat and keep within a healthy weight range.

- Dairy foods such as full-fat Greek yogurt and whole milk can be beneficial for the prevention of obesity and metabolic syndrome.

- Supplementing with high linoleic acid safflower oil, CLA, and fish oil can be a valuable combination in the fight against obesity.

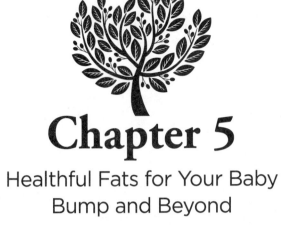

Chapter 5

Healthful Fats for Your Baby Bump and Beyond

I can honestly say my greatest accomplishment has been the birth of my two precious sons, Luca and Matteo. They truly are the light of our world, and I feel so blessed and honored to be their mom. I was lucky; my pregnancies were easy —as far as pregnancies go—very little to almost no morning sickness, moderate weight gain, no acne. Yep, my boys were kind to me. My deliveries, however, were a bit more challenging, and I have to admit that being a new mom was quite overwhelming for me, something that I think all my friends who had done this before me forgot to mention. Being awake during the night, learning how to nurse a hungry baby, dealing with the crying, and then the feeling of having lost part of my identity, admittedly, left me feeling guilty and as though I were the worst mom in the world. It's funny how scared I was to tell my family that I was feeling like this, especially after the birth of my first son, Luca. Like many moms, I went from enjoying a rewarding career, doing yoga when I pleased, going for walks and hikes alone, and quality time with my husband, all with no mommy guilt, to suddenly finding myself tethered to home with a fussy baby, not even having enough time to shower in the day, while my husband ventured out to work in his suit for a day full of meetings, lunches, and, well, peace.

But I quickly began to learn some of the lessons of motherhood—to expect the unexpected, to revel in a new way of life, and humility (yes, childbirth has a way of doing that). Once Luca settled, or perhaps I settled, I really did start to enjoy it. Although I still found being a mom the most rewarding and loving experience, it was the hardest thing I have ever done. Nevertheless, I let myself have fun. I spent hours on the floor with blocks and toys, puzzles and books. I enjoyed making his baby food, nursing him, bathing him, and rocking him to sleep. But, most definitely, the best feeling ever in my life has been the bond I feel with my two sons. Being able to provide the unending, selfless gift of life and love is what I have learned from them. I am a better person because of my boys.

I write this chapter about the importance of nutrition for you and your baby with a ton of love and experience. My boys are my passion in life, and there is nothing I wouldn't do for them. They are surrounded with love, health, and goodness, and my goal is to raise them to be confident, loving, positive children of God. All we can do as parents is help show them the way, and hope they don't venture too far off the path we have laid down for them.

Another goal as moms is to teach our children how to eat, nurture, and respect their bodies so they will enjoy a lifetime of health. We are the drivers, the teachers, and the role models for our children when it comes to healthful eating. They will learn and follow what we do. Therefore, we must start nurturing them with the best nutrition possible, even before we conceive. The healthier we are during pregnancy, the healthier our children will be. This chapter is dedicated to Luca and Matteo and the incredible love I have for them and the respect I hold for mothers everywhere.

Eating for Two

Everyone requires omega-3s and omega-6s, but the need is crucial during pregnancy and lactation. Increased omega nutrition is required during pregnancy for the proper development of the mammary glands, placenta, and uterus, and for the development of the fetus, especially during the last trimester of pregnancy, when the fetus absorbs the greatest amounts of healthful fats. Fetal energy and nutrient demands result in a 50 percent or higher increase in maternal requirements for omega-3s and omega-6s. Omega-3 fatty acids are actively transported across the placenta, which is how all nutrients are supplied to the fetus. Large amounts of the omega-3 fatty acid DHA pass through the placenta, which is the most abundant fatty acid in the brain, retina, and neuronal tissue. Deposition of DHA starts in the second half of pregnancy with the estimated accumulation in the fetal brain of approximately 76 mg per day by the third trimester. For this reason, premature babies are more vulnerable to an omega-3 deficiency; they may not have had enough time to absorb adequate fats.

"Eating for two" should be your mantra with regard to consuming healthful fats, not only during pregnancy but also if you are trying to get pregnant. The diet before pregnancy plays an important role in determining maternal omega-3 status. Because omega deficiency is so commonplace, boost your intake beforehand in anticipation of the extra nutritional requirements during pregnancy. Research shows that after four weeks of essential fatty acid (EFA) supplementation, tissue levels of DHA increased significantly.[1]

In a study published in the *British Journal of Nutrition*, researchers tested the hypothesis that maternal supplementation during the second and third trimesters of pregnancy enriches maternal and/or fetal DHA status. One hundred mothers received either fish-oil capsules containing 400 mg of DHA or a placebo from fifteen weeks' gestation until term. The study found that maternal DHA status was maximal in mid-trimester and declined to term at a lower rate in supplemented compared with nonsupplemented mothers. The researchers concluded that maternal DHA supplementation significantly increases maternal DHA status and limits the last trimester decline, aiding preferential transfer of DHA from mother to fetus.[2]

Fetal DHA and arachidonic acid (AA) needs are extremely high during the last trimester because 70 percent of brain-cell development takes place while the fetus is in the womb.[3] The fetal liver is not mature enough to be able to metabolize shorter-chain fatty acids into the long-chain omega-3s and is unable to supply them until sixteen weeks after birth. Therefore, to obtain sufficient levels of omega-3s, the fetus depends on the transport of fatty acids from the mother across the placenta. Pregnant women need adequate omega-3s for their own needs as well as for the growing baby (although the mother's requirements for her own body tend to decrease during pregnancy, which is nature's way of allowing the growing fetus to have sufficient supply). If the pregnant woman is depleted of omega-3s before pregnancy, neither the mother nor the baby will have an adequate quantity of healthful fats for brain, retina, immune system, and nervous system development.

DHA may be the most critical EFA, because women deficient in DHA may deliver preterm as well as low-birth-weight babies or experience postpartum depression.

Omega-3s for Longer Gestation and Higher Birth Weight

Every year over 13 million babies are born prematurely around the world. It is important to identify modifiable causes of preterm delivery, which is a strong predictor of an infant's later health and survival. From the cognitive standpoint, a longer period of gestation affords the developing fetus more time for the central nervous system to develop. There is evidence that Inuit populations, such as those from the Faroe Islands, with a high fish intake have longer gestation periods, larger babies, and reduced incidences of pre-eclampsia (pregnancy-induced high blood pressure) compared with those populations who consume less fish.

A study published in *The Lancet* showed that mothers on the Faroe Islands gave birth to bigger babies than those born in Denmark, partly due to longer gestation periods.[4] This observation is supported by data from a study where supplementation with omega-3 fatty acids (2.7 g/day) from the thirtieth week of the pregnancy was associated with increased gestation (four days) and higher birth weight (107 g heavier) compared with the control group receiving olive oil as a supplement.[5]

Fish oil has been shown in randomized trials and animal experiments to have the potential to delay spontaneous delivery and prevent preterm delivery, but the minimum amount of omega-3 fatty acids needed to obtain this effect remains to be determined. Researchers from Denmark set out to investigate these issues in a study of 8,729 women whose seafood intake in early pregnancy was assessed by a questionnaire. They tested whether a low intake of seafood in early pregnancy was a risk factor for preterm delivery and low birth weight and whether it was associated with a lower fetal growth. The group found that 1.9 percent of women who ate fish at least once a week had a premature birth, but this increased to 7.1 percent among women who never ate fish. The researchers concluded that low consumption of fish was a strong risk factor for preterm delivery and low birth weight.[6]

However, pregnant women should know that there is increasing evidence of mercury and other heavy-metal poisoning in our fish supply, and if they are consuming fish, they should either omit certain fish during pregnancy or reduce their intake to once every couple of weeks unless they know the source of the fish. The safest way to consume omega-3 fatty acids without the risk of heavy-metal poisoning is to consume high-quality fish oil supplements that have been tested for mercury and other heavy metals and comply with industry standards for safe levels. The Environmental Protection Agency is a reputable source for information on mercury and fish consumption.[7]

Expert groups have recommended 200 to 300 mg EPA plus DHA per day during pregnancy (these are very conservative dosages because they are based on general recommendations for healthy adults).

Table 1: Expert Committee DHA and EPA Intake Recommendations during Pregnancy*

Expert Group	Daily DHA Recommendations
European Commission	200 mg
International Society for the Study of Fatty Acids and Lipids	300 mg
National Institutes of Health	300 mg
World Association of Perinatal Medicine	200 mg

Sources: Artimis P. Simopoulous, Alexander Leaf, and Norman Salem Jr., "Workshop Statement on the Essentiality of and Recommended Dietary Intakes for Omega-6 and Omega-3 Fatty Acids," *Prostaglandins, Leukotrienes & Essential Fatty Acids* 63 (September 2000): 119–121.

Hania Szajewska, Andrea Horvath, and Berthold Koletzko, "Effects of n-3 Long-Chain Polyunsaturated Fatty Acid Supplementation of Women with Low-Risk Pregnancies on Pregnancy Outcomes and Growth Measures at Birth: A Meta analysis of Randomized Clinical Trials," *American Journal of Clinical Nutrition* 83 (June 2006): 1337–1344.

Good Fish, Bad Fish

The current, 2004, FDA recommendations continue to recommend up to two fish meals per week. In May 2010, nutritional experts petitioned the commissioner of the FDA to change the wording of the current advisory to indicate that women should eat *at least two* servings of fish per week, noting that maximal benefits may involve consumption over 12 ounces (340 g) per week. The FDA recently completed an extensive analysis of the risks of methylmercury and the benefits of consuming fish during pregnancy and concluded that eating fish has a significantly higher net benefit on childhood development than adverse effects from possible prenatal mercury exposure.[8] The Institute of Medicine reconciles these views by stating that the benefits of eating fish are greater than not eating fish, as long as pregnant women consume low-mercury fish.[9]

No serious side effects have been reported in pregnant women taking fish oil supplements in clinical trials—other than an increase in belching and an unpleasant taste noted by some women.

Table 2: Safe and Unsafe Fish during Pregnancy*

Fish to Avoid	Safer Fish to Eat
Fresh tuna	Grouper
King mackerel	Halibut
Shark	Lobster
Swordfish	Canned light tuna
Snapper	Wild salmon
Tilefish	Trout

*Source: Department of Health and Human Services, US Food and Drug Administration, "Mercury Levels in Commercial Fish and Shellfish (1990–2010)," May 26, 2011, accessed December 5, 2009, http://www.fda.gov/Food/FoodSafety/Product-SpecificInformation/Seafood/FoodbornePathogensContaminants/Methylmercury/ucm115644.htm?utm_campaign=Google2&utm_source=fdaSearch&utm_medium=website&utm_term=Mercury Levels in Commercial Fish and Shellfish&utm_content=1.

Because DHA and EPA stay in the bloodstream for some time, a 200 to 300 mg per day average can be obtained by eating two 6-ounce (170 g) servings of high omega-3 fish per week. Oily fish are typically deep cold-water fish and are also good sources of vitamins A and D. The most common sources are salmon, tuna, mackerel, and sardines. These are fish that have oils throughout the entire fillet rather than only in the liver, as is typical of cod, for example. Omega-3s are also found in plant foods (please see chapter 2 for more information on food sources). But remember, as discussed in chapter 1, these plant sources need to be converted into EPA and DHA before they can be used by the body, brain, and, subsequently, the infant. Therefore, ideally, oily fish should be the primary source of omega-3s during pregnancy, along with a high-quality omega-3 supplement (please see the resources section on page 193 for quality brands). Fish consumption is also a healthful protein source and a great alternative to red meat, which makes this food-based approach for omega-3s superior.

When choosing fish, many people forget that canned fish can be a great option; for example, canned salmon and canned tuna are wild and less expensive than their "fresh" counterparts, but still a very nutritious option for omega-3s. Light tuna packed in water can be eaten twice per week, whereas canned white albacore should be limited to once per week because it is higher in mercury, although it is still within safe limits.[10,11] For salmon, always choose wild Alaskan salmon over farmed salmon (all Atlantic salmon is farmed) giving a much higher count of the chemical pollutant polychlorinated biphenyl (PCB). Trim away the fatty areas of the salmon before cooking to reduce PCB intake. For more information on wild versus farmed salmon, please see chapter 7, as well as the Association of Reproductive Health Professionals' guidelines.[12]

Table 3: DHA and EPA Content in Food*

Food		DHA (mg per 6 oz / 170 g serving)	EPA (mg per 6 oz / 170 g serving)
Salmon			
	Atlantic salmon, farmed	2,477	1,173
	Atlantic salmon, wild	2,429	699
	Chinook salmon, farmed	1,236	1,717
	Coho salmon, farmed	1,481	694
	Canned sockeye salmon	1,190	901
Other Fish			
	Sardines (3.75 oz / 106 g can)	468	435
	Atlantic herring (3 oz / 85 g)	939	773
	Pickled herring (1 cup / 250 mL)	746	843
	Farmed catfish	653	250
	Atlantic/Pacific halibut	636	154
	Canned light tuna	1,137	240
	Flounder/Sole	439	413
	Rainbow trout, farmed	1,394	568
	Atlantic cod	262	7
Shellfish	Alaskan king crab	602	1504
	Dungeness crab (1 crab)	144	357
	Blue crab (canned, 1 cup / 250 mL)	230	261
	Shrimp	245	291
Other	DHA-enriched eggs	130–150/egg	0

*Source: US Department of Agriculture, National Agricultural Library, "Nutrient Data Laboratory," May 16, 2012, accessed June 4, 2012, http://www.ars.usda.gov/main/site_main.htm?modecode=12-35-45-00.

Fish for Brawny Brains

I know every mother and father wants to do what they can to ensure their child has the best head start for school. I love the fact that numerous studies have supported the benefit of omega-3s for mothers while they are pregnant—for the developing fetus, and then for children as they grow. The first few months after birth, the central nervous system rapidly develops, and during this phase of rapid growth, the brain is sensitive to a lack of nutrients. An adequate supply of omega-3s, especially DHA, is necessary for maintaining optimal tissue during this time. Normal visual and cognitive development is dependent on this supply due to the central structural role of DHA. A study in 2007 showed that infants from mothers who supplemented with DHA during pregnancy had significantly improved visual acuity at four and six months of age.[13]

Clinical trials have showed low childhood IQ scores and visual function in healthy term infants due to a lack of DHA and AA in the diet.[14] A study published in the *American Journal of Clinical Nutrition* found that pregnant women who ate more fish gave their babies a better chance at mature brain development. The study also found that mothers with more DHA in their blood had babies with better sleep patterns in the first forty-eight hours following delivery compared with those mothers who consumed less fish.[15] It has been hypothesized that infant sleep patterns reflect the maturity of a child's nervous system, and are associated with more rapid development in the first year of life. The omega-3 DHA, along with the omega-6 arachidonic acid (AA), is the key building blocks for healthy brain and eye development.

DHA is extensively incorporated into the placenta and is the most abundant fatty acid in the brain, retina, and neural tissue. DHA starts to be deposited during the second half of pregnancy, with the estimated accumulation in the fetal brain of approximately 76 mg of DHA per day in the third trimester.[16] Prenatally, DHA is obtained from maternal stores, whereas postnatally, it is obtained from breast milk or infant formula. In a clinical trial called the "DIAMOND Study," a total of 181 infants were enrolled at one to nine days of age and assigned to receive one of four term infant formulas with different levels of DHA and arachidonic acid. The infants received the formula for twelve months. Cognitive function was assessed in 131 children at eighteen months of age using the Bayley Scales of Infant Development. This study is of particular importance because it is the first to evaluate cognitive outcomes in infants assigned to multiple DHA levels found in formula. The scientists concluded that supplementation of DHA during the first year of life leads to enhanced cognitive development at eighteen months of age.[17]

In the last few years, research has centered on increasing the omega-3 supply to the fetus by supplementing the mother's diet with omega-3s. Multiple studies have reported higher DHA levels in cord blood at birth of children born to supplemented women compared with those whose mothers did not receive DHA supplements during pregnancy.[18,19,20] The issue of the mother receiving DHA supplementation on brain development of their children remains controversial. Some studies report better performance on different neurological examinations by children whose mothers received supplements during pregnancy, but others did not show that much effect. However, I was very impressed by a study published in the *Journal of Nutrition* in 2011 that examined prenatal DHA status and neurological outcome in children at age 5.5. The scientists compared healthy pregnant women from Spain, Germany, and Hungary who were randomly assigned to a dietary supplement consisting of either fish oil (500 mg DHA + 150 mg EPA), 400 mg 5-methyltetrahydrofolate, both, or placebo from twenty weeks gestation until delivery. The odds of children with the maximum neurological optimality score (NOS) increased with every unit increment in cord blood DHA level at delivery. Therefore, higher DHA levels in fetal and maternal blood during the course of pregnancy were related to better performance on neurological exams of children 5.5 years of age.[21]

Baby Blues

Within four days after delivery, the mother's tissue demands for nutrients such as the omega-3s are several times those of the pregnant uterus before term. In fact, recent research confirms that 700 to 800 mg of DHA is taken up by the breast milk in the first three months postpartum, and the mother supplementing in the second half of pregnancy results in increased DHA and EPA levels in breast milk.[22] This finding is significant regarding the health benefits for the infant. At this time, no studies have reported on the effect of omega-3s on the quantity of milk or the duration of breast-feeding. If the mother is not consuming enough DHA, then deficiencies in DHA may be especially apparent postpartum. DHA status declines during pregnancy, especially during multiple pregnancies, with levels normalizing slowly, probably within one year postpartum. In fact, it can take up to four years to replace the DHA that is transferred to the fetus during pregnancy. This is why it is imperative that pregnant women supplement with fish oil. I recommend at least 1,000 mg of EPA + DHA combined. (Please see the resources section on page 193 for recommendations.)

A mother's DHA needs to remain high not only during pregnancy but also during lactation. Research finds women with low levels of DHA may be at an increased risk of developing a condition known as postpartum blues, which has been shown to progressively worsen with each successive pregnancy.

Approximately 15 to 20 percent of women who give birth in the United States develop postpartum depression. Dr. Joseph Hibbeln, director of the Mother and Child Foundation of the National Institutes of Health, has studied the effects of fish consumption and risk of postpartum depression. He concluded that countries with higher fish consumption, such as Japan, Hong Kong, Sweden, and Chile, had the lowest levels of postpartum depression, whereas countries with the lowest fish consumption (South Africa, Germany, and Saudi Arabia) had the highest rates of postpartum depression.

Omega-3s Are Baby Fuel

Lactating women have an increased need for DHA, since breast-fed babies require a constant supply. As previously mentioned, up to 800 mg of DHA are taken up by the breast milk during the first three months postpartum. While omega-3s are critical for the development of a healthy fetus, they are equally important as the infant grows and matures. Human breast milk is 50 percent fat, which is the fuel for the tremendous rate of growth in newborn infants. While breast milk has been known as the perfect food for an infant because of its nutritional and biological properties, the proportion of DHA and other omega-3s in breast milk varies from population to population. Numerous studies have found that the content of DHA in mother's milk depends largely on the type and quantity of food consumed.[23] Research has shown that breast milk of women living in Canada and the United States is deficient in omega-3s in comparison with women in China and Japan. Canadian and European studies have confirmed that pregnant women do not ingest the amount of omega-3s needed. Dietary changes to increase consumption of healthful fats during pregnancy and lactation should be a primary goal for women.[24]

Breast Milk Omega-3s

DHA
DPA
EPA
ALA

0   0.5   1   1.5

■ American
□ Chinese
■ Japanese

While the long-term consequences of inadequate levels of omega-3s are not completely understood, research supports the observations that infants who are lacking in omega-3s have lower visual acuity and are at greater risk of developing attention-deficit disorders (ADD and ADHD) and depression later on in life. Remember, the retina of the eye has the largest concentration of DHA over any other part in the body, making DHA an extremely valuable component for healthy vision.

Dietary Concerns with Obtaining DHA and EPA

- North American women typically do not eat enough seafood.

- Nineteen percent of Americans eat the recommended two servings of fish per week.

- Women with low financial resources are more likely to have a diet low in DHA and EPA compared with women with greater resources.

- Valid concern about potential fetal-toxic effect from fish consumption.

- Many oily fish high in omega-3s are predators, and being higher in the food chain, they are, therefore, more likely to contain contaminants such as PCBs; methylmercury (a well-known neurotoxin) and PCBs are considered endocrine disruptors associated with reduced fertility and certain cancers.

- In May 2010, nutritional experts petitioned the FDA to change the current advisory to indicate women should eat at least two servings of fish per week, noting that maximum benefits may involve consumption of over 12 ounces (340 g) per week. The FDA recently completed an extensive analysis of risks of methylmercury and the benefits of consuming fish during pregnancy and has concluded that eating fish has a significantly higher net benefit on childhood development than adverse effects from possible mercury exposure.

Omega-3s for Strong Immune Systems

There are three groups of nutrients that I believe to be critical for the development of a healthy immune system in your baby. First of all, breast-feeding (albeit challenging at first, but so important) gives your baby valuable colostrum (especially during the first few days), which research proves is full of healthful antibodies needed by the baby to develop a strong immune system.

Second is probiotics (healthful bacteria), which are naturally found in mother's milk. When babies come into this world through a vaginal delivery, they actually gain beneficial bacteria through the vaginal tract that helps to develop the good bacteria inside their digestive tracts. And thirdly, but of equal importance, healthful fats, especially DHA and EPA, which promote immune-cell development by acting as a substrate for antibodies involved in modulating allergic inflammatory responses.

Numerous studies positively associate higher omega-3 levels in cord blood with subsequent reduction in the development of childhood allergic diseases, such as asthma, autoimmune disease, atopic dermatitis, and allergic rhinitis.

DHA is strongly linked to the regulation of allergic responses and immune-system control. Research has linked higher prenatal DHA intake to a number of positive developmental outcomes in both infants and children.[25]

Fish Oil Helps Combat Antibiotic-Induced Asthma in Preschool Children

Antibiotic treatment in early life has been shown to increase the risk of future allergic disease, asthma, autoimmune conditions such as psoriasis, and even colds and influenza. We know that *antibiotics* (the Greek word for "anti-life") destroy all bacteria in the gastrointestinal (GI) tract, good and bad, which leaves us with a compromised digestive system. Eighty percent of our immune system is found in our GI tract; therefore, if the bacteria become imbalanced in favor of the bad, it opens us up for all kinds of health issues. Swedish scientists have shown an increased risk of wheezing in infancy following antibiotic exposure during the first week of life.[26]

We know that because omega-3 fatty acids and certain omega-6s such as gamma-linolenic acid (GLA) can influence the development of allergic disease by acting in a positive way on inflammatory and immunological pathways, the introduction of fish oil would seem to be a wise choice. Upon the early introduction of fish, researchers have noted a beneficial effect on the risk of eczema in infancy, and on allergic rhinitis at preschool age, not to mention the beneficial effect of preventing asthma.[27] I love it when I read research that supports this, and then I also hear hundreds of moms share their stories about how omega-3s have changed their kids' lives.

Omega-3s from fish oil should be introduced under nine months of age and continued for essentially the rest of our lives. Omega-3s along with probiotics are, in my opinion, the two most important nutrients to supplement the diet. *My recommendation is for approximately 500 mg of EPA and DHA per day for kids under twelve. For twelve and older, I recommend a minimum of 1,000 mg of EPA and DHA per day.*

Quality Checks for Supplements

When choosing supplements, products should be based on purity and on the amount of EPA and DHA in the product, not on the total amount of fish oil. The amount of DHA and EPA will vary with each brand. While supplements can be a simple way of increasing omega-3s, there is significant variation in supplement quality. This is one of the reasons I have partnered with the International Fish Oil Standards (IFOS) for my brand of fish oils. IFOS is a Canadian-based organization that has initiated a voluntary program to examine supplement purity and to provide objective information to consumers and providers in evaluating supplement quality. Care must be taken to store fish oil in a cool environment because exposure to high temperatures can cause fatty acids to lose their double bonds and structure. (Please see the resources section on page 193 for information about SeaLicious.)

Behavioral and Learning Disorders: The Omega-3 Connection

Childhood should be a special time filled with fun and excitement. Although this may be true for many children, more and more are being diagnosed with behavioral problems (keeping in mind that children are supposed to be energetic and full of life). However, when a child's energy pulls them from one task to another in a blink, and you notice your child is unable to concentrate, becomes bored with activities quickly, and is always looking for something else to do, then a behavioral problem may be present. These children tend to perform poorly in an academic environment. Children can be classified as hyperactive, aggressive, or a combination of both. These conditions can be classified as attention-deficit disorder (ADD) or attention-deficit/hyperactivity disorder (ADHD). ADHD is being identified as an epidemic, affecting 5.29 percent of school-age children (these are the documented and diagnosed cases) all over the world, and functional impairment persists in up to 70 percent of all affected children through adulthood.[28] ADHD is more common in young boys than in young girls.[29] The exact cause is not known; however, many factors interact to cause the problem. Why have we seen such a dramatic increase in these learning and behavioral difficulties in our children? I don't remember any of my friends having these issues when I was a child. Now it is commonplace. Is it a difference in diagnosing or labeling them, or are we so much more sophisticated in our knowledge? The significant change in our diet that has occurred over the last twenty years, in particular the high consumption of sugar and decrease in healthful fats are major indicators for what we are seeing today. We have witnessed as much as a four to five times increase in children being diagnosed with these conditions. This is why we see improvements in the symptoms when diet changes are implemented.

Research has suggested a strong nutritional link between abnormalities in cell communication and cognitive and behavioral disturbances associated with autism, ADD/ADHD, dyslexia (reading and writing disorders), dyspraxia (coordination and developmental disorders, where the coordination of motivation and action is problematic), oppositional behavioral disorders, and impaired social behavior, as well as anxiety and tic disorders.[30]

Research has shown that a relative lack of omega-3 fatty acids, in addition to high omega-6 (too much arachidonic acid) creates an imbalance that can lead to ADHD and other neurodevelopmental disorders. Another focus of research has been whether or not there is an increased need for certain fats, such as DHA, in some individuals.[31] DHA has been recognized for its importance in learning, memory, and concentration. Laura J. Stevens suggests in a study published in the *American Journal of Clinical Nutrition* that an altered fatty acid metabolism is a key contributor to the nutritional deficiencies in children with behavioral and learning disorders. The fifty-three study participants with ADHD had lower concentrations of EFAs in their blood cells compared with forty-three controls.[32]

The same researchers continued their studies on young boys with learning disorders. They found a greater number of behavior problems, temper tantrums, learning disorders, and sleep difficulties in the participants with lower total omega-3 concentrations. The efficiency in which omega-3s are metabolized is lower in boys than girls due to gender differences and the influence of testosterone. This is one of the reasons why autism, ADD, and ADHD are higher in boys than girls.[33]

EFA Combination Improves Learning Disabilities

A study published in *Progress in Neuropsychopharmacology and Biological Psychiatry* in 2002 examined the effects of EFAs on ADHD-related symptoms in children with specific learning disabilities (mainly dyslexia). Forty-one children ages eight to twelve years with specific learning difficulties and above-average ADHD ratings were randomly allocated to the EFA supplementation group for twelve weeks. After twelve weeks of EFA supplementation, improvements were noted in attention, restlessness-impulsiveness, anxiousness-shyness, and cognitive problems. The researchers concluded that EFA supplementation appears to reduce ADHD-related symptoms in children with dyslexia.[34]

Other researchers, such as Dr. Jacqueline Stordy, have had success with a combination of fish and evening primrose oils. Stordy said that children who consume enough EFAs become calmer and their reading skills improve.[35] In another study, Richardson and Puri observed a decline in cognitive disorders and general behavioral abnormalities and psychosomatic symptoms such as anxiety, shyness, cognitive problems, inattentiveness, hyperactivity, and impulsiveness. Supplementing with DHA and EPA in combination with AA and GLA led to a decline in numerous symptoms.[36]

One of the most impressive studies I have read is called the "Oxford-Durham Study," in which a supplement comprising fish oil and evening primrose oil was tested for its effectiveness on the abnormal behavior of children with dyspraxia. Of the sixty children in the active treatment group, fifty-five exhibited significant reading/writing weaknesses, and fifty had pronounced ADHD symptoms, whereas all fifty-seven children in the placebo group had considerable reading/writing difficulties, and fifty-two had pronounced ADHD symptoms. The supplement of an EPA, DHA, and GLA mixture resulted in significant improvements in the reading/writing difficulties and ADHD symptoms, as well as the aggressive and anxious behavior. At the end of the thirty-month treatment, clinically relevant ADHD symptoms were evident in only 23 percent of all children.[37] I find this to be compelling, exciting, and utterly amazing. As I have said before, if we give our bodies the ability to heal, they can with the proper food and nutrients.

Omega-3s Can Help Autistic Children

Autism spectrum disorders usually become noticeable after age two and into early childhood. They are characterized by social interaction and communication weaknesses, as well as by stereotypical behavior. Children often display behavioral abnormalities such as self-harm, aggression, and fits of rage. However, children suffering from autism also possess strength in perception and attention, as well as memory and intelligence. The moderate success of the drugs used to treat autism is often disproportionate to their deleterious side effects.[38] As is the case with ADHD, dyslexia, and dyspraxia, it has become clear that autism spectrum disorders are also related to a deficiency of omega-3s. For example, children with autism show lower amounts of omega-3s in their blood compared with healthy children. One study involving 861 autistic and 124 healthy children established a relationship between the low DHA and AA levels in infant formula and the occurrence of autism. Babies receiving infant formula low in DHA and AA are at a much greater risk of developing autism spectrum disorders than children who are breast-fed.[39]

In another study investigating omega-3 supplementation on autistic children, the parents reported a general improvement in the health of their children. The children were able to sleep better and concentrate more easily, and they displayed improved cognitive and motor abilities and were more sociable and less irritable, aggressive, and hyperactive.[40]

Summary of Omega-3 Benefits for Children's Health

- Improved sight/vision
- Improved central nervous-system functioning
- Improved IQ
- Greater ability to concentrate, focus
- Healthier sleep patterns
- Improved motor abilities
- More sociable and less irritable, aggressive, and hyperactive
- Stronger immune systems
- Reduced risk of asthma and allergies
- Less anxiety
- Decreased risk of ADHD, dyslexia, dyspraxia, and autism spectrum disorders
- Greater motor skills

Summary of Omega-3 Benefits for Pregnant Women

- Greater maternal stores to supply the fetus via the placenta
- Greater supply of breast milk

- Reduced risk of postpartum depression
- Healthy skin, hair, and nails
- Stronger immune system (less illness during pregnancy)
- Longer gestation; carry to term
- Bigger babies

Table 4: Effects of Omega-3 Fatty Acids on Neuronal Mechanisms*

Mechanism of Action
Cerebral development
Development of vision
Component in neuronal membrane phospholipids
Effects on neurotransmitter systems
Regulation of corticotrophin-releasing hormone
Inhibition of protein kinases
Modulation of heart-rate variability
Improved cerebral circulation and oxygen supply
Prevention of neuronal apoptosis
Influence on energy exchange
Influence on neurite growth
Regulation of gene expression
Anti-inflammatory effects

*Source: Marlene P. Freeman, Joseph R. Hibbeln, Katerine L. Wisnder, et al., "Omega-3 Fatty Acids: Evidence Basis for Treatment and Future Research in Psychiatry," *Journal of Clinical Psychiatry* 67 (December 2006): 1954–1967.

How to Get Our Kids to Eat Good Food

You may be compelled by some of the data that I presented in this chapter to make a few changes in your kids' diets to favor healthful fats and less sugar. Yes, I agree, it is easier said than done, especially for your picky eater. As a mom, I have tried my best to instill healthful nutrition into our lives. In fact, at a recent birthday party my four-year-old told the hostess that he wanted only a little cake because he didn't want to eat that much sugar. Yes!

Incorporate These Mom-Proofed Tips

- The earlier you start the better. This begins right from the introduction of solid food. Start with vegetables before fruit to allow their taste buds to learn the blander, less sweet taste. Even though current recommendations say it doesn't matter, I think it does. It is more challenging to enjoy green peas after a banana, especially if you don't understand the nutritional benefit of the peas.

- We are their best role models. And by this I mean what we eat, they are sure to follow. For us, it starts with the grocery shopping. I know that if we buy packaged "treats," they will get eaten, which is why I try to keep them to a minimum. Instead, I always try to have on hand string cheese, yogurt (Greek yogurt is a favorite), fresh fruit, cut-up vegetables (which are a bit more difficult for kids under two years of age), whole-grain crackers, natural nut butters, and healthful whole-grain cereals. Kids seem to like to graze, eating all day. If they have healthful food to graze on, then it shouldn't be a problem.

- No juice. And I mean none. It just isn't necessary. If they don't get used to drinking juice, they won't know what they are missing. In my opinion, juice provides mostly sugar, and although it does have vitamins and minerals (in orange juice), it is better to cut up an orange and give it to your kids as a whole food. Milk (or a dairy alternative) and water should be the main sources of hydration.

- If you give them something new once and they don't like it, try it again. It could take up to ten times of introducing a food before they like it.

- Enhance the flavor of food. When I steam broccoli, I always toss in a clove of garlic and a pinch of sea salt, and then when it's cooked, I drizzle the broccoli with olive oil. My boys love it. I wouldn't want to eat bland-tasting broccoli either, but there are many ways to make it taste yummy.

- Introduce fish as early as you can. I started my boys on white fish when they were around eight months of age. It is their most preferred protein source. Lightly sautéed with grapeseed oil, salt, lemon, and garlic, they would choose this for dinner over anything else.

- Minimize packaged food. Again, if you don't buy it, you won't eat it. Leave packaged food for emergency situations. We need to get back to cooking as a family. Your kids will love the activity of buying groceries and preparing food. I know it can be a bit stressful, and certainly not quick, yet I promise it will be worth your effort. And if you aren't able to do this every night, then try it at least two times per week. This will help to instill healthful nutrition as you will be able to explain why we need to eat certain foods.

- Start fish oil supplementation at a young age (around one year). Fish oils have come a long way in taste and palatability. Most liquid fish oils on the market are naturally sweetened and flavored, making them taste quite delicious. My boys have been using fish oils since they were six months old, and in fact always want "more" than the allotted ½ teaspoon (2.5 mL).

What You Have Learned in This Chapter

- Prenatal nutrition is of utmost importance to the development of the fetus, in particular omega-3 fatty acids.

- What we put into our kids is what we get out, including time, love, energy, and nutrition. This I speak to from experience.

- Instill healthful habits by being the best role model you can be. Your kids will eat what you eat.

Chapter 6

Healthful Fats for a Healthy Heart

When you look down the aisles of your neighborhood grocery store, you can see why cardiovascular disease is the top killer in Canada and the United States. Ninety percent of the products on the supermarket shelves are highly processed foods that are rich in unhealthful fats, loaded with sugar, and depleted of fiber. Combine these foods with lifestyles marked by inactivity, sleep deprivation, and stress, and you create a constellation of physiological phenomena that include low levels of good cholesterol (HDL), high levels of harmful triglycerides, and high blood pressure.

Cardiovascular disease (CVD), namely heart disease and stroke—continues to reign as the number one cause of death in Canada and the United States. One in four Canadians has some form of heart disease—about 8 million people. About 60 million Americans suffer from heart disease. Yet this is a "lifestyle disease" that can be largely prevented by not smoking, making healthful choices, increasing physical activity, and maintaining a healthy weight.[1] This means that if we change our environment we can reduce the likelihood of developing disease. So why, if we know we can prevent CVD, as well as type-2 diabetes and obesity, and even certain types of cancers, are they still the top chronic diseases that people are dealing with?

DNA Is Not Destiny

When my husband and I were traveling to Bora Bora for our ten-day honeymoon back in 2006 (where does time go?), I was adamant that all BlackBerrys, laptops, and other modes of communication be left at home so that we could disconnect and enjoy a restful and recharging honeymoon. However, I did say that novels and magazines were allowed. I bought *InStyle* and an assortment of gossip magazines (my guilty pleasure and escape from reality); my husband bought *Time* and *Discover Magazine*. (Yes, you can see the differences in our personalities just from our magazine choices.) Fortunately, the issue of *Discover Magazine* my husband picked up had a profound article that demonstrated that DNA is not destiny.[2] Dr. Morello, my husband, has now shared this information with thousands of people at countless lectures, and I know it really hits home for many people. In the article, the author described two distinctly different individuals—one who was taller and larger than the other. These two people also had different facial features. Yes, even though it appeared as if these two were unrelated, the shocking fact was that they were identical twins. Essentially, identical twins are supposed to be carbon copies of each other, yet these two were far from identical. So what happened? When the scientists studied this anomaly, they discovered that these men had been separated at birth and grew up in two very different environments. The foods they ate, the water they drank, the air they breathed, and the nurturing they received were all different—and it was these differences that changed the behavior of their DNA.

DNA Is Not Destiny discussed how the environment can affect the body's ability to read DNA. This may eventually prove that the reason some people develop cancer, heart disease, diabetes, eczema, Alzheimer's disease, and a host of other diseases isn't that they inherited these conditions, but rather that they live in the same environment their parents did and mimic their behavior.

Fats Can Change Our Cells

In chapter 1, I discussed how essential fatty acids are the building blocks of cells and that, essentially, a diet full of bad fats leads to bad cell structures, which in turn can be linked with depression, cardiovascular disease, immune-system impairment, joint pain, diabetes, and obesity—and the list continues.

Of all the areas studied with respect to omega-3s and disease prevention, there is no area that shines brighter than that of healthful fats for a healthy heart.

Cholesterol Crazy

Cholesterol is the most misunderstood subject in nutrition. Cholesterol for some reason has received the most attention. In fact, it is often a measurement by which people judge their overall health. A conversation goes like this: "So what did the doctor say? How are you?" "Well, my cholesterol is normal, so I am good." Cholesterol is found in the bloodstream and in every cell in your body. Cholesterol is used to form cell membranes and is needed to produce sex hormones, such as estrogen, androgen, and progesterone, and adrenocorticoid hormones, as well as to manufacture vitamin D. Of the cholesterol in the blood, 75 percent is produced by the liver. Most people have a feedback mechanism that moderates their cholesterol levels. For a small group of people, however, their cholesterol-regulating system in the liver is dysfunctional and their cholesterol levels must be maintained by making changes in their diet.

Transporters

Lousy Cholesterol: LDL

Cholesterol is transported in the blood in various protein components known as lipoproteins, including low-density lipoprotein (LDL), high-density lipoprotein (HDL), intermediate-density lipoprotein (IDL), and very-low-density lipoproteins (VLDL). These transport proteins vary in their effects on the body. If too much LDL cholesterol circulates in the blood, it can slowly build up on the lining of arterial walls. This condition is known as atherosclerosis (hardening of the arteries). A clot that forms near this plaque can block the blood flow to part of the heart muscle and cause a heart attack. This is why LDL cholesterol is called the bad, or lousy, cholesterol. Also, when the LDL particles are small and dense, it can further lead to a heart attack. The American Heart Association recommends that our LDL cholesterol be less than 2.6 mmol/L (100 mg/dL).[3]

How to Lower LDL Levels:

- If you are in the moderate- to high-LDL cholesterol range, that is, 3.3 mmol/L (130 mg/dL) or higher and you have coronary heart disease, or 4.9 mmol/L (190 mg/dL) and you do not have coronary heart disease, then medication may be required to initially bring levels down into the safe zone.

- Numerous studies show that lifestyle changes such as exercise, smoking cessation, weight loss, and following a heart-healthy diet can reduce cholesterol levels, and thus the risk of heart disease.

- Eat heart-healthy foods. These include avocados, almonds, garlic, shiitake mushrooms, oat bran, legumes and beans, onions, fatty cold-water fish, ground flaxseeds, and extra virgin olive oil.

- Take natural supplements such as omega-3 fatty acids from fish oil, resveratrol, garlic, beta-glucans, polymethoxylated flavones, vitamin B6, coenzyme Q10 (CoQ10), and hydroxy citric acid.

Happy Cholesterol: HDL

Research shows that HDL cholesterol tends to carry cholesterol away from the arteries and back to the liver for disposal. HDL acts like a bottom-feeder in a fish tank. It cleans off the walls of the blood vessels, thus removing excess LDL cholesterol. HDL cholesterol is known as "good" cholesterol because a high level of HDL seems to protect against heart attacks. Even small increases in HDL cholesterol reduce the frequency of heart attacks. For each 0.03 mmol/L (1 mg/dL), or 1 percent, increase in HDL cholesterol, there is a 2 to 4 percent reduction in the risk of coronary heart disease.

To Increase HDL Levels:

- Regular cardio exercise (aerobic exercise) that burns between 1,200 and 1,500 calories each week can have dramatic results.

- By losing ten pounds of excess weight (fat), you will see a significant increase in HDL cholesterol.

- If you smoke, quit—cigarettes decrease HDL cholesterol levels. A study published in *Preventive Medicine* showed that HDL cholesterol levels increased by approximately 4 mg/dL (0.12 mmol/L) following smoking cessation.[4]

- Lower your carbohydrate intake (especially processed, refined, white carbs). Avoid everything white: white bread, white rice, white sugar, white flour, white potatoes. Studies prove that HDL levels drop dramatically when blood sugar is spiked by carbohydrates.

- Take natural supplements such as GLA, EPA + DHA (from fish oil), fiber supplements, and tons of antioxidants such as resveratrol and CoQ10.

A news report shows that only 13 percent of US adults have high total cholesterol, which is very interesting, especially since CVD is still the number one killer in the United States, a country where two-thirds of adults are overweight.[5] The reason cited was that so many Americans use cholesterol-lowering drugs, yet if the prevalence of cholesterol has decreased, why are rates of heart disease still so high?

The old "cholesterol hypothesis" suggested that elevated cholesterol in the blood increases the risk of CVD, and that a high intake of saturated fat increases blood cholesterol. This theory is completely outdated and far too simple. In fact, we know that our diet is missing a healthful level of good saturates (short- and medium-chain), and this deficiency is one of the factors related to an increased risk of CVD and metabolic syndrome. It's important to remember that cholesterol is only one of 200 risk factors for heart disease, meaning there are other factors that are far more important to consider. As well, cholesterol-lowering drugs have numerous side effects, decreasing levels of coenzyme Q10 being one of them—this is linked to heart attacks and heart disease, which could be one of the possible explanations for low cholesterol yet high rates of heart disease.

Triglycerides

Triglycerides are a storage form of fat. They come from the food we eat and from the fats produced by the body. Fatty acids get stored as triglycerides, as do excess sugars and refined carbohydrates. Our bodies have a limited capacity to use sugar, so once it reaches that capacity, the sugar gets converted into fat and stored as a triglyceride. During the low-fat, no-fat diet craze in the 1980s and 1990s, many people were eating low-fat food products that were loaded with sugar. During this time, triglyceride levels soared. This is why we need to eat only those carbohydrates that can be burned. Elevated triglyceride levels are positively associated with an increased risk of heart disease.

To Lower Your Triglyceride Levels

- Cut back on simple sugars such as juice, soda, cookies, and candy, along with table sugar, sweeteners (including artificial sweeteners), honey, and syrups (high-fructose corn syrup).

- Reduce carbohydrate-containing foods such as bread, pasta, white rice, and white flour. Instead, think about fibrous carbohydrates only.

- Obesity is a major cause of high triglycerides. If you are overweight, lose weight and exercise.

- Use natural supplements. Fish oils shine with respect to lowering triglycerides. The American Heart Association recommends 2 to 3 grams of omega-3s per day.

Recommended Cholesterol Levels*

- Total Cholesterol: Less than 200 mg/dL (5.1 mmol/L)

- LDL Cholesterol: Less than 100 mg/dL (2.56 mmol/L)

- HDL Cholesterol: Women: Greater than 50 mg/dL (1.3 mmol/L)

- Men: Greater than 40 mg/dL (1.0 mmol/L)

- Triglycrides: Less than 150 mg/dL (1.7 mmol/L)

Source: Expert Panel on Detection, Evaluation, and Treatment of High Blood Cholesterol in Adults, "Executive Summary of the Third Report of the National Cholesterol Education Program (NCEP)," *Journal of the American Medical Association* 285 (May 2001): 2486–2497.

Obesity and Heart Disease

Carrying excess weight, especially in the abdominal region, is a risk factor for heart disease. (Please see chapter 4 for more on this relationship.) Being overweight increases your risk of high blood pressure. In fact, blood pressure rises as body weight increases. Losing even ten pounds can lower blood pressure, and it has the greatest effect for those who are overweight and already have high blood pressure.

The Nurses' Health Study found that the risk of developing coronary artery disease increased three to four times in women who had a body mass index (BMI) greater than 29. A normal BMI should be between 19 and 24. A Finnish study showed that for every 1-kilogram (2.2 lb.) increase in body weight, the risk of death from coronary artery disease increased by 1 percent. In patients who have already had a heart attack, obesity is associated with an increased likelihood of a second heart attack.[6]

How to Reduce Your Risk of Heart Disease

Dietary and lifestyle interventions are critical to the management of abnormal blood lipids. The following changes should be considered:

- Reduce trans fats
- Exercise at least thirty minutes per day
- Reduce salt in your diet
- Increase consumption of antioxidants
- Eat fewer simple sugars; focus on fibrous food
- Limit alcohol consumption
- Reduce stress
- Use natural supplements, especially omega-3s from fish oil, and take antioxidants such as CoQ10 and resveratrol

Heart-Friendly Flax

Fish and its corresponding omega-3s, EPA and DHA, have received much positive attention for their heart-health benefits, which might leave vegetarians feeling as though they are out of luck. However, flaxseed and other plant sources of the omega-3

ALA, such as camelina oil, are extremely beneficial for the heart. The Mediterranean-style diet (rich in olive oil, tomatoes, and fish), which is high in both plant and fish omega-3s, can reduce the incidence of sudden death by 70 percent after two years. A study that compared the cholesterol levels in Crete, Greece, and Zutphen, Netherlands, reported the Cretans had higher concentrations of ALA and lower cholesterol levels than the Dutch. ALA in the Cretan diet comes from purslane, walnuts, and other wild dark green leafy plants.

The National Heart, Lung, and Blood Institute Family Heart Study examined the relationship between ALA-rich omega-3 oils and coronary artery disease. More than 4,500 participants filled out food-frequency questionnaires, and the results of the study showed that a higher intake of ALA and LA had a synergistic effect on the risk of developing coronary artery disease, with higher intakes of ALA and LA corresponding to lower risks.[7]

And one of the most significant landmark studies examining the relationship between dietary ALA and heart disease was the Nurses' Health Study. The dietary habits of more than 120,000 registered nurses were followed for more than ten years. Nurses with the highest dietary intake of ALA experienced 30 percent fewer fatal heart attacks than those who consumed lower amounts of ALA.[8] Regular consumption of ground flaxseeds and/or flaxseed oil would provide similar results.

Chia Seed: Ancient Seed, but New Kid on the Block

I have been incorporating ground flaxseeds into my diet for almost fifteen years. The health benefits are enormous. However, I love to have a balanced and varied diet, which is why I was excited to learn of another great plant source of omega-3s, fiber, and protein: chia seed. It's interesting to note that the word "chia" is derived from the Nahuatl word *chian*, which means "oily." Although not a new seed, it has become known as one of the top superfoods that people should consume.

My first memory of chia is from the TV commercial that had the catchy tune of "cha, cha, cha, cha, cha, cha chia," which went on to advertise the little Chia Pet clay animals with sprouted chia seeds covering their bodies. As a child, I had no idea that those tiny seeds provided such tremendous nutritional value and medicinal properties.

In a small recent study on postmenopausal women, 25 grams/day of ground chia seed over a seven-week period resulted in significant increases in blood levels of ALA and EPA, which offers numerous health benefits for heart health.[9] In another study on individuals with metabolic syndrome, subjects consumed chia seed and saw improvements in their body weight and waist circumference, as well as decreases in their triglyceride and fasting blood sugar levels. Chia seed's abundance of protein, healthful fats, and tons of fiber make it an excellent food choice for those with heart disease, type-2 diabetes, or metabolic syndrome, and those who are overweight.[10]

Recommendation for Plant-Based Heart Health

Consume 2 tablespoons (30 mL) of ground flaxseeds or chia seeds per day. They are very easy to incorporate into all foods, including smoothies, yogurt, soups, cereals, bread, hot dishes, pasta sauce, and almost every other food. Just ensure the flaxseeds and/or chia seeds are ground to receive all the nutrition from the seed, or for a more convenient option, you can buy them already ground.

Fishing for Heart Health

Over the past few decades, an impressive number of studies have shown that fish is good for the heart. Research has shown that omega-3 fatty acids decrease the risk of arrhythmias (abnormal heartbeats), which can lead to sudden death. Omega-3 fatty acids also decrease triglyceride levels, slow the growth rate of atherosclerotic plaque, and lower blood pressure (slightly). In 2000, the American Heart Association (AHA) released dietary guidelines recommending everyone consume at least two servings of fatty fish per week to protect against heart disease. The AHA then updated their guidelines, stating that for patients with coronary artery disease, at least 1 gram of omega-3s per day is recommended. Similarly, for those with elevated triglyceride levels, 2 to 3 grams of omega-3s per day is desirable. This is a major milestone and the first time an organization such as the AHA has endorsed supplement use. The AHA realized the recommended dosages may be greater than what can be readily achieved through diet alone.

Table 1: Potential EPA and DHA Benefits*

Antiarrhythmic effects
Improvements in autonomic function
Decreased platelet aggregation
Vasodilation
Decreased blood pressure
Anti-inflammatory effects
Improvements in endothelial function
Plaque stabilization
Reduced atherosclerosis

Reduced free fatty acids and triglycerides
Upregulated adiponectin synthesis
Reduced collagen deposition

Source: Carl J. Lavie, Richard V. Milani, Mandeep R. Mehra, and Hector O. Ventura., "Omega-3 Polyunsaturated Fatty Acids and Cardiovascular Diseases," *Journal of the American College of Cardiology* 54 (August 2009): 585–594.

The 1970s' Great Fish Find

In the late 1970s, two Danish scientists, Dyerberg and Bang, were the first to highlight the cardio-protective effect of dietary omega-3 fats found in fatty fish in the Inuit population.[11] Over the past thirty years, the mechanisms by which fish oils improve cardiovascular health have been extensively studied, showing anti-inflammatory, antiarrhythmic, and antiaggregatory effects, as well as improvements in endothelial function.

Fish Oil Lowers Inflammation

We have all heard that an aspirin a day keeps the doctor away, especially for those with heart disease. The reason aspirin is so effective at decreasing heart attack risk has to do with its ability to thin blood, and also its anti-inflammatory benefits. Upon the action of aspirin, EPA and DHA can be converted by the COX and LOX pathways (please see chapter 1) into similar families of resolvins, E and D series, which have tremendous anti-inflammatory benefits for heart health. The role of chronic inflammation in the diseases that modern society is now dealing with has become far-reaching, and the influence of nutrition and dietary impact serious.[12] Most studies have shown a correlation between diet and markers of inflammation called "C-reactive protein (CRP)," a protein produced by the liver when arteries become inflamed. In a study published in the journal *Circulation*, women who had the highest CRP levels were two times more likely to have a cardiovascular event.[13] In chapter 4, I discussed the science of high linoleic safflower oil and its ability to reduce CRP levels by 17.5 percent in women who were obese, post menopausal, and type-2 diabetic.

A traditional Mediterranean diet pattern rich in olive oil, tomatoes, fish, and an abundance of fruit and vegetables, legumes, and grains, can provide tremendous anti-inflammatory benefits.

Because fish oil is rich in omega-3 fatty acids, research has shown its ability to decrease inflammatory markers such as CRP. A study involving 130 people with metabolic syndrome each received 1,000 mg of fish oil daily over a six-month period. These individuals saw a significant reduction in CRP levels, cholesterol, and triglycerides.[14] Omega-3s from fish oil is an important dietary strategy for managing heart disease risk factors caused by excessive inflammation.

Fatty Fish Lowers Cholesterol and Triglycerides

Triglycerides—the blood storage form of fat (which is increased by not just fat, but by too much sugar in our diet as well),— are a major risk factor for heart disease, possibly even greater than high total cholesterol. Luckily, this is where fish oils shine in their ability to reduce triglyceride levels by 30 to 40 percent when using approximately 4 grams of EPA and DHA daily.[15] The results are very effective, even in comparison with some pharmaceutical drugs. The US Food and Drug Administration (FDA) has approved an omega-3 PUFA formula at a dosage of 4 grams/day for the treatment of very high triglyceride levels

(> 500 mg/dL).[16] This dose has been shown to reduce severely elevated triglyceride levels (> 500 mg/dL) by 45 percent, along with reduction in non-high-density lipoprotein cholesterol by 14 percent with a 9 percent increase in high-density lipoprotein cholesterol.[17] When added to statin therapy in patients with triglyceride levels between 200 and 499 mg/dL, this dosage of omega-3 PUFAs lowers triglyceride levels by close to 30 percent.[18] A dose-dependent relationship exists for fish oil and triglyceride-lowering: The higher the doses used, the greater the reduction in triglyceride levels.

Research shows that as triglyceride (TG) levels increase, so do the number of coronary heart events.[19] The mechanism in which they lower TG is complex; however, we know that they regulate the expression of genes that encode the key proteins controlling the metabolism and formation of very-low-density lipoproteins carrying triglycerides in the liver.[20] Omega-3s also reduce the formation of triglycerides by the liver.

Fish Reduces Heart Palpitations

Arrhythmias (abnormal electrical conductivity of the heart that causes irregular heart beats) is a serious risk factor for heart attacks. There is strong clinical evidence suggesting the cardioprotective role of fish oil, which is significant because there is currently no pharmaceutical drug treatment for arrhythmias. Dr. Alexander Leaf, professor of clinical medicine at Harvard Medical School, commented in the journal *Circulation*, "Animal studies show that fatty acids from omega-3 fish oils are stored in the cell membranes of heart cells and can prevent sudden cardiac death or fatal arrhythmias."[21] Dr. Leaf said that studies of individual heart cells demonstrate that omega-3s specifically blocked excessive sodium and calcium currents in the heart, which can cause dangerous and erratic changes in heart rhythm.[22] On examining the effects of different toxic agents on heart cells, they observed that adding omega-3s prevented arrhythmias induced in the cells. In a large study of 5,096 men and women, a high fish intake was associated with a lower heart rate and slower atrioventricular conduction.[23] Recent research has started to focus on DHA's role in the prevention of arrhythmia over EPA, with knowledge that there is a greater amount of DHA than EPA in the heart muscle. According to doctors, at least half of all heart attacks are caused by irregular heartbeats.

Fish Oil Reduces Heart Attack Risk

Some of the most impressive research comes from heart studies showing the benefit of fish on reducing sudden cardiac death. We know that the risk of dying from a heart attack goes up exponentially in people who have already suffered one. There have been three large randomized trials that have documented the effects of omega-3s in primary and secondary prevention of coronary heart disease. For example, the Diet and Reinfarction Trial (DART) was the first clinical trial to evaluate the effects of omega-3s on survival. DART included 2,033 men who were recruited in twenty-one British hospitals an average of forty-one days after having a heart attack. The people in this study were divided into groups and given advice to receive either a lower-fat diet, increasing fatty fish intake to at least two fish meals per week (200 to 400 grams of fatty fish per week), or fish-oil capsules and increasing fiber intake. After two years, the group that was advised to increase their fatty fish intake had an impressive 29 percent reduction in deaths from any cause, but mainly due to a reduction in fatal heart attacks. The reduction in heart attacks was particularly impressive in the group who consumed fish-oil capsules as opposed to simply increasing dietary fish consumption.[24]

More recently, two major randomized trials were performed. The infamous GISSI (Gruppo Italiano per lo Studio della Sopravvivenza nell'Infarto Miocardico)-Prevenzione study, which divided the 11,323 patients (who had suffered a heart attack within the past three months) into four different groups:

- Group 1: Patients received 1 gram of fish oil (containing 85% EPA and DHA in a ratio of 1.2:1)
- Group 2: Patients received 300 mg of vitamin E
- Group 3: Patients received a combination of fish oil and vitamin E
- Group 4: Control group (patients did not receive anything)

The results were very significant for dietary supplementation with omega-3s from fish oil. Treatment with omega-3s resulted in an impressive 45 percent reduction in the risk of having a sudden fatal heart attack, a 30 percent decrease from heart-related death, and a 20 percent reduction in overall death.[25]

In another trial, the JELIS (Japan EPA Lipid Intervention Study) trial, in which 18,645 patients (14,981 in primary prevention, 3,664 in secondary prevention) with high cholesterol (70% women) were divided into groups to receive either statin alone or statin with fish oil containing the high level 1,800 mg/day of EPA. At the end of the five-year study, those in the EPA group had a 19 percent reduction in major cardiovascular events.[26]

Krill Oil Is Good for the Heart

Krill oil first came to my attention in 2004 as the new kid on the block for omega-3s. It has a unique profile in that the omega-3s

EPA and DHA are found in their phospholipid structure, which enhances their absorption. Not only that, but krill is known as a super antioxidant from its rich astaxanthins. It has greater antioxidant potential than CoQ10 and vitamin E. Krill is also known as "whale food" and is a shrimp-like crustacean with a bright red color (from the rich astaxanthins). However, we don't have to worry about depleting the supply of whale food because there are maximum allowable fishing limits set for krill-catching to ensure it stays sustainable. The majority of krill is caught off the coast of Antarctica.

I have seen many people use krill oil with great success in the area of heart health and PMS. (I have many female friends who found relief from their PMS symptoms with krill over any other natural product they tried.)

There are a few stand-out clinical trials with respect to krill oil. One of them assessed the effects of krill oil on blood lipids, specifically total cholesterol, triglycerides, low-density lipoprotein (LDL), and high-density lipoprotein (HDL). Over a period of three months, 120 patients were given the following:

- Group A: Krill oil at a BMI-dependent daily dose of 2 to 3 grams daily
- Group B: 1 to 1.5 grams of krill oil daily
- Group C: Fish oil containing 180 mg of EPA and 120 mg of DHA per gram of oil at a dose of 3 grams daily
- Group D: A placebo

The researchers found that 1 to 3 grams per day of krill was effective for reducing blood sugar, triglycerides, LDL, and HDL compared with both fish oil and placebo. It was significantly more effective than even fish oil for overall blood lipid improvements.[27]

Summary of American Heart Association Recommendations[28]

- Eat fatty fish (salmon, mackerel, lake trout, sardines, albacore tuna, and halibut) at least two times per week; 3.5 ounces (100 g) cooked, or about ¾ cup (185 mL) of flaked fish

- Patients with coronary heart disease: 1,000 mg of EPA and DHA per day

- Elevated triglycerides: 2,000 to 4,000 mg of EPA and DHA per day

Table 2: Fish Content of EPA and DHA*

Type	DHA (g/100g)	EPA (g/100g)	DHA and EPA (g/100g)
Bluefin tuna	1.141	0.363	1.504
Light tuna, canned in water	0.223	0.047	0.270
Albacore tuna, canned in water	0.629	0.233	0.862
Atlantic salmon, farmed	1.457	0.690	2.147
Atlantic salmon, wild	1.429	0.411	1.840
Chinook salmon	0.727	1.010	1.737
Sockeye salmon	0.700	0.530	1.230
Atlantic mackerel	0.699	0.501	1.203
Atlantic herring	0.699	0.504	1.203
Rainbow trout, farmed	0.820	0.334	1.154
Rainbow trout, wild	0.520	0.468	0.988
Halibut	0.374	0.094	0.465
Cod	0.154	0004	0.158
Haddock	0.162	0.076	0.238
Channel catfish, farmed	0.128	0.049	0.177
Channel catfish, wild	0.137	0.100	0.237

Swordfish	0.681	0.087	0.768
Grouper	0.213	0.035	0.248
Shrimp	0.144	0.171	0.315

*Source: Carl J. Lavie, Richard V. Milani, Mandeep R. Mehra, and Hector O. Ventura, "Omega-3 Polyunsaturated Fatty Acids and Cardiovascular Diseases," *Journal of the American College of Cardiology* 54 (August 2009): 585–594.

Summary of Food Strategies to Improve Heart Health

1. Limit intake of trans fats and red meat (one to two servings of red meat are suggested per week). Try to cut any excess fat from meat, or choose leaner cuts.

2. Increase consumption of fatty fish (at least two servings per week).

3. When choosing culinary oils, use heart-healthy extra virgin olive oil for salad dressings and as a garnish. Use coconut oil, avocado oil, or camelina oil for medium- to high-heat cooking.

4. Increase consumption of dietary fiber. Fiber helps to mop up extra cholesterol from the blood, helps to balance blood sugar, provides a feeling of fullness, and helps shed extra weight.

5. Enjoy your food baked or grilled and fry less often (when you do fry, make sure to match your oil with the smoke point and cooking application; please see chapter 3).

6. Choose low-sodium seasonings such as spices, herbs, and lemon juice in cooking and at the table.

7. Increase consumption of antioxidant-rich foods (remember, antioxidants help to deactivate and absorb all the free radicals that damage cellular walls). Consume

foods such as berries, dark green leafy veggies, citrus fruit, green tea, and red wine.

8. Eat fewer simple sugars; focus on fibrous carbohydrates only.

9. Limit alcohol consumption (other than the occasional glass of red wine, which is loaded with heart-healthy resveratrol).

10. Increase consumption of anti-inflammatory foods, especially turmeric.

11. Exercise at least thirty minutes per day, five days per week.

12. Use natural supplements such as omega-3s from fish or krill oils.

What You Have Learned in This Chapter

- Heart disease is largely preventable with proper diet and lifestyle strategies.

- Omega-3 fatty acids from fish oil and krill oil are highly effective strategies for the reduction of total cholesterol and triglyceride levels.

- Ground flaxseeds and chia seeds can be easily added to all foods and provide the diet with fiber, omega-3s, and protein, nutrients that are known to improve heart health.

Chapter 7

The Full-Fat Solution Nutrition Tips

The nutrition you put in your mouth each day is the single most important factor in achieving a healthy body. After you read this book, I hope you no longer feel frightened about incorporating healthful, nutritious fats into your diet. I promise, you will not gain weight, and, if anything, you will be surprised by how lean your body looks; how shiny and healthy your skin, hair, and nails are; how much better you are able to concentrate; and how much more energy you have when you start incorporating real food into your diet. We need to get our food back to the way nature intended.

Some Important Eating Principles

1. Get in the habit of planning your meals in advance so you don't need to go to the grocery store every day.

2. Choose recipes that are relatively easy and quick and save the more labor-intensive ones for weekends and special occasions. You can create healthful food quickly.

3. Eat fatty fish at least two times per week. I have many delicious recipes using salmon and halibut.

4. When possible, eat wild fish.

5. Canned fish is a nutritious, economical option (please see the resources section on page 193 for recommended brands).

6. Eat a protein, fibrous carbohydrate, and healthful fat with each meal and snack.

7. Eat five or six small meals per day.

8. Have an assortment of cooking and garnishing oils available.

9. Consume Greek yogurt, preferably plain; flavor it yourself with fruit.

10. Consider a variety of dairy alternatives such as rice milk and almond milk to achieve different flavors, tastes, and textures.

11. Invest in a juicer and/or blender as a way to create delicious and healthful smoothies.

12. Make small changes to avoid overwhelming yourself. Small changes will lead to a lifetime of healthful eating. Remember, I didn't always juice spinach and kale and love it. This has come over a decade of making changes to my diet to benefit my health.

Nutritious Staples to Keep in Your Pantry and Refrigerator

There are a few staple foods that I recommend everyone keep on hand or, if produce, to buy weekly in order to create healthful, delicious meals. When you can, purchase organic and free-range meat and eggs. Special recipes usually require some planning ahead to make sure you have all the necessary ingredients. In fact, if on

Sunday you can plan your meals for the week, it will save you time, money, and stress as you will be prepared with ideas and supplies. Try to cook enough food to last at least for lunch the next day or as leftovers for another family dinner. However, the following checklist will ensure you have enough healthful ingredients on hand to prepare a healthful dinner for your family.

Canned and in Jars

- An assortment of beans (cannellini, black, chickpeas, lentils)
- Fish (salmon and tuna) (Please see the resources section on page 193 for a recommended brand.)
- Natural nut butters (including tahini, peanut butter, and almond butter)
- Tamari sauce
- Tomatoes (stewed, whole, diced)
- Vinegar (balsamic, red wine, white wine, rice)

Dry

- Couscous
- Dried fruit (sulfite-free mangos, apricots, prunes, coconut flakes, dates)
- Hemp hearts
- Jasmine, basmati, brown, and wild rice
- Nuts and seeds (almonds, hazelnuts, cashews, sunflower seeds, pumpkin seeds, flaxseeds, chia seeds)
- Pasta (a variety of types; whole wheat is preferable)
- Quinoa
- Sprouted-grain bread
- Steel-cut oats
- Whole-wheat flour

Frozen

- Berries (strawberries, blueberries, raspberries)
- Fish and seafood (cod, halibut, other white fish, prawns)
- Meat (buy fresh, then package in small freezer bags; chicken: boneless, skinless breasts, and thighs)
- Vegetables (corn, peas, mixed)

Fresh

- Asparagus
- Avocados
- Bananas
- Beets
- Bell peppers
- Blueberries
- Broccoli
- Carrots
- Celery
- Cilantro
- Garlic
- Kale
- Lemons
- Limes
- Mixed greens (including baby spinach, arugula)
- Potatoes
- Romaine lettuce
- Shallots
- Strawberries
- Yellow and red onions

Culinary Oils

- Camelina oil
- Coconut oil
- Extra virgin olive oil
- Grapeseed oil
- Organic flaxseed oil
- Safflower oil

Spices and Herbs

- Basil
- Cracked pepper
- Garlic
- Greek seasoning
- Oregano
- Rosemary
- Sea salt
- Thyme

Refrigerated

- Butter
- Cream (10% and 33%)
- Dairy milk (including rice, almond, hemp, cow's)
- Eggs
- Greek yogurt (plain)
- Hard cheese (asiago, Parmesan, Cheddar, feta)

A Word about Farmed versus Wild Fish

I thought it was important to discuss eating wild fish instead of farmed because I am often asked what kind to buy, Atlantic or Pacific, fresh or canned. There is a lot of chatter and discussion on the Internet about this hot topic. For me, the most important consideration is the accumulation of toxins that are found in fish farms, which subsequently are found in the meat of the fish.

In 2004 in the journal *Science*, researchers warned about farmed salmon because of the unacceptably high levels of the pollutants polychlorinated biphenyls (PCBs) and dichlorodiphenyltrichloroethane (DDT) that concentrate in the good fat.[1] These compounds are traced back to the salmon feed, and although they have been banned for decades, they biodegrade slowly and linger in the water and soil. And when they accumulate in the body, they increase the risk of cancer, metabolic syndrome, insulin resistance, type-2 diabetes, and immune-system dysfunction.[2] Unfortunately, a more in-depth look at these chemicals is outside the scope of this book, but please see the recommended reading list on page 191 for more information on this important topic.

What Is Fish Farming?

The aquaculture industry (known as fish farming) involves raising fish in pens, some of which are open to the ocean. Fish farms are known as cesspools for toxins because of the amount of chemicals and antibiotics used to control disease. The most common species raised by fish farms are salmon, European sea bass, catfish, cod, carp, and tilapia.[3] With that being said, since the publication of the study in the journal

Science in 2004, fish-feed manufacturers cleaned up their act with cleaner feed, and governments began to regulate contaminants more stringently. Ruth Salmon, head of the Canadian Aquaculture Industry Alliance has been quoted saying, "We have improved vaccines with which we treat our young fish and antibiotic use has dropped dramatically in the past years; we are comfortable that we have good management practices for fish health."[4]

Omega-3 Content

Each type of salmon contains different amounts of fat, and remember, the fat is where the omega-3s are found.

Table 1: Nutrition Profile of Omega-3s per 3.5 Ounces (100 g) of Uncooked Meat*

Salmon Type	Omega-3 (g)
Pacific coho	0.95
Atlantic, farmed	1.4
Pacific chinook	1.9
Pacific chum	0.81
Pacific sockeye, fresh	2.7
Pacific sockeye, canned	2.9
Pacific pink, fresh	1.3
Pacific pink, canned	2.4

**Source*: Agriculture and Agri-Food Canada, "Fish and Seafood: Fact Sheets," December 2007, accessed June 6, 2012, http://www.ats-sea.agr.gc.ca/sea-mer/fhs-eng.htm.

The most common wild Pacific salmon are chinook or king; coho or silver; sockeye or red; chum, or keta, or dog; and pink. Canned salmon is an excellent option, and it is mostly wild because it is from British Columbia and Alaska. Atlantic salmon is always farmed. Following are the four most common salmon species that you will find in your grocery-store seafood department.

Chinook (also known as King, Spring, and Tyee)

This is the largest of the wild Pacific salmon. Chinook offers an array of rich flavors. Their flesh is soft, big, and flaky. Chinooks are the fattiest of the three salmon species, which makes them high in the omega-3s EPA and DHA. They are best grilled as a whole fish or on planks, or smoked or baked. This is my personal favorite, and I find it to be the easiest to serve to guests because it does not impart as "fishy" a flavor as the other varieties.

Coho

Coho are very versatile with rich, full flavors. This fish does very well with minimal garnish or seasoning; its firm flesh is ideal for grilling.

Sockeye

The smallest of the four, sockeye are an incredibly strong species because they swim against strong currents. Known for their unique flavor, this fish can be best described as "wild." Sockeye are excellent grilled as fillets or steaks, baked, planked, smoked, or poached.

Wild Pink

Wild pink salmon is the most abundant salmon species in the Pacific Ocean. Pinks have the mildest flavor, low oil content, and a small flake. Most pink salmon is canned because it is considered trash, yet it is actually the cleanest of species from a pollutant standpoint. If purchasing fresh or frozen pink salmon, use preparation methods such as marinating beforehand or cooking with moist heat methods so as not to dry the meat out.

Agriculture and Agri-Food Canada offers excellent information on fish farming and wild fish as well as the life-cycle of fish. Please see the resources section on page 193 for their website, where you can find fact sheets on a variety of fish and seafood.

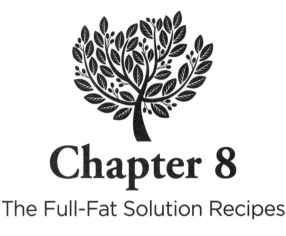

Chapter 8

The Full-Fat Solution Recipes

I am very excited to share some of my favorite recipes that incorporate healthful fats. Developing nutritious recipes that everyone can easily create at home is an intensive process, but it is a labor of love. I am lucky to have amazing friends, family members, and professionals in my life who helped make these recipes a reality by providing suggestions, taste-testing, and encouraging the process. These full-fat recipes are a small sample of many more that I will be sharing in my upcoming e-recipe book, *The Full-Fat Solution Recipe Book*. You might note that I do not provide the nutrition information for these recipes because I want you to enjoy your food without worrying about calories. Each of these recipes is clean and contains wholesome, nutritious ingredients. My dream is for everyone to enjoy them.

As the Italians say, "Buon appetito!"

Nutty Strawberry-Spinach Energy Elixir

This is one of my favorite ways to start the day. It provides tons of nutrition and energy for on the go!

Yield: 4 servings

　　2 cups (500 mL) rice milk or beverage of your choice
　　1 banana
　　8 frozen strawberries
　　3 cups (750 mL) packed baby spinach leaves
　　¼ cup (60 mL) raw cashews
　　1 tablespoon (15 mL) ground flaxseeds
　　1 teaspoon (5 mL) organic flaxseed oil

Combine all the ingredients in a Vitamix or other blender or food processor and blend until smooth. Enjoy!

Flax-Berry Blast

Protein shakes became a staple in my diet in 2004, and I can honestly say they are a foundation in my health plan to this day. I have made every version of protein shake you can imagine, but this one is the most popular among my friends and family.

Yield: 1 to 2 servings

　　1 scoop (0.9 ounces / 25 g) vanilla whey protein (I like whey
　　　　protein isolates or organic whey)
　　1 cup (250 mL) berries of your choice, fresh or frozen
　　1 teaspoon (5 mL) ground flaxseeds
　　1 cup (250 mL) your favorite beverage (water, whole milk,
　　　　rice or almond milk, but favor the original varieties over
　　　　the flavored ones to avoid extra sugar)

Combine all the ingredients in a blender or food processor and blend until smooth.

Variations: Vary this recipe by changing the type of fruit, milk beverage, or protein powder flavor.

Peanut Butter–Banana Smoothie

This recipe combines my two favorite foods—peanut butter and chocolate. Does it get any better than this?

Yield: 1 to 2 servings

> 1 scoop (0.9 ounces / 25 g) chocolate whey protein powder (either organic whey or whey protein isolate)
> 1 tablespoon (15 mL) natural peanut butter or almond butter
> ½ banana (not overly ripe)
> 1 cup (250 mL) organic whole milk or beverage of your choice
> 1 teaspoon (5 mL) ground flaxseeds
> Ice cubes (optional)

Place all the ingredients in a blender or food processor and blend until smooth.

Creamy Scrambled Eggs

My boys and I usually eat organic free-range eggs each morning. Eggs are really the perfect protein, and they help to provide a necessary source of protein first thing in the morning. This easy, yet so creamy and delicious recipe will certainly become a favorite breakfast item for your family.

Yield: 2 servings (to serve more people, double or triple the recipe)

> 2 organic free-range eggs
> 1 tablespoon (15 mL) organic cream (10% milk fat)
> 1 tablespoon (15 mL) ricotta cheese
> Pinch of sea salt
> Pinch of cracked black pepper
> 1 teaspoon (5 mL) butter
> ½ avocado, sliced

Crack the eggs into a small glass bowl. Add the cream, cheese, salt, and pepper. Beat with a fork until light and fluffy.

Melt the butter in a small skillet over low heat (do not overheat, otherwise the butter will burn). Pour the egg mixture into the pan, and allow it to slightly cook before stirring with a wooden spoon. Cook until the scrambled eggs are done to your liking.

Divide between two plates and garnish with the slices of avocado. Serve with sprouted-grain toast for a nutritious and delicious breakfast.

Monkey Pinwheels

My boys really love this combination of natural hazelnut spread and bananas. These are great as a quick snack or breakfast on the go.

Yield: 2 servings

> 1 tablespoon (15 mL) organic hazelnut spread
> (I particularly like Green & Black's)
>
> 1 tablespoon (15 mL) natural almond or peanut butter
>
> 1 (10-inch / 25 cm) whole-wheat tortilla
>
> 1 banana

Spread the hazelnut spread and then the almond butter on the tortilla. Slice the banana overtop. Roll up the tortilla, slice it into small pieces, and serve.

Papaya-Avocado Salad ▬▬▬▬▬▬▬▬▬▬

I first tried this recipe at a girls' night over a decade ago, and it has stuck with me ever since. I have since modified a few of the ingredients, but it's a summertime favorite!

Yield: 6 servings

Salad:

> 1 head of butter lettuce or mixed lettuce, washed and dried
> 1 ripe papaya (papayas are ripe when they have turned yellow)
> 1 large avocado, peeled and sliced
> Red onion slices, as many as you like

Papaya-Seed Dressing:

> ¼ cup (60 mL) organic cane sugar
> 2 tablespoons (30 mL) papaya seeds (from the papaya above)
> 2 teaspoons (10 mL) sea salt
> ½ teaspoon (2.5 mL) dry mustard
> ½ cup (125 mL) white wine vinegar
> ½ cup (125 mL) your favorite salad oil

Tear the lettuce into bite-size pieces, and put in a salad bowl. Halve and peel the papaya, and scoop out the seeds, saving 2 tablespoons (30 mL) for the dressing.

To make the dressing, combine the dressing ingredients in a food processor and blend until the papaya seeds have the appearance of ground pepper.

Just before serving, add the papaya, avocado, and red onion slices to the lettuce. Pour your desired amount of dressing over the salad. Leftover dressing can be stored in an air-tight container in the fridge.

Greek Salad

Greek salad is one of my favorites. I love this recipe served with chicken or lamb, or on those nights when I just feel like a salad and some fresh bread—delicious!

Yield: 4 to 6 servings

Dressing:

  ½ cup (125 mL) extra virgin olive oil
  3 tablespoons (45 mL) red wine vinegar
  1 teaspoon (5 mL) freshly squeezed lemon juice
  ½ teaspoon (2.5 mL) sea salt
  ½ teaspoon (2.5 mL) oregano
  Freshly cracked black pepper to taste

Salad:

  ½ cucumber, quartered lengthwise and diced
  2 tomatoes, cut into large chunks
  ½ red onion, thickly sliced
  1 red bell pepper, chopped
  1 orange bell pepper, chopped
  ½ cup (125 mL) chopped pitted black Kalamata olives
  Feta cheese, crumbled or cubed, as much as desired
  Sprinkle of sea salt
  Sprinkle of dried oregano

To make the dressing, combine all the dressing ingredients in a jar with a tight-fitting lid and shake well.

To make the salad, combine the cucumber, tomatoes, onion, bell peppers, olives, and cheese in a salad bowl. Just before serving, pour the dressing overtop, sprinkle with the salt and oregano, and toss gently.

Nutty Pear and Brie Salad

My best friend, Tamara, introduced me to this recipe, and I loved the taste of the Brie cheese and pear together. I usually favor organic Bosc pears in this salad for an extra-flavorful, crunchy treat. You can also choose to candy the walnuts by boiling maple syrup, mixing it with walnuts, and then baking them at 400°F (200°C) for a few minutes until candied.

Yield: 6 to 8 servings

Dressing:
> ¼ cup (60 mL) extra virgin olive oil
> ¼ cup (60 mL) white wine vinegar
> 2 tablespoons (30 mL) apple juice
> 2 tablespoons (30 mL) Dijon mustard
> 1 garlic clove, minced
> ½ teaspoon (2.5 mL) sugar

Salad:
> 2 Bosc pears
> 8 cups (2 L) torn salad greens (your choice of arugula, spinach, butter lettuce, and romaine lettuce)
> 4 ounces (125 g) cold Brie cheese, cubed
> 1 cup (80 mL) chopped pecans or walnuts
> ½ cup (125 mL) chopped green bell pepper

To make the dressing, combine all of the dressing ingredients in a glass jar with a tight-fitting lid or in a shaker cup. Shake to mix well. (Leftover dressing can be refrigerated; remove at least 1 hour before using because the olive oil will solidify in the fridge.)

To make the salad, put the salad greens in a large serving bowl and sprinkle the cheese, nuts, and bell pepper over the lettuce. Toss with the dressing just before serving.

Flaxseed Oil Dressing

This dressing is delicious served over your favorite salad.

Yield: about ¾ cup (185 mL)

> ½ cup (125 mL) extra virgin olive oil
> ¼ cup (60 mL) flaxseed oil
> 3 tablespoons (45 mL) red wine vinegar
> 1 garlic clove, minced
> 1 teaspoon (5 mL) dry mustard
> 1 teaspoon (5 mL) Parmesan cheese
> 1 tablespoon (30 mL) Italian herbs
> Salt and pepper to taste

Put all the ingredients in a jar with a tight-fitting lid, and shake well. Pour over a salad and toss. Store in the fridge. If you refrigerate this dressing, remove it at least 1 hour before using so the olive oil has a chance to return to its original liquid state.

Best-Ever Guacamole

I absolutely love the flavor of guacamole and could eat it on everything, from eggs to crackers, nachos, potatoes, and many fish recipes, especially halibut tacos. Guacamole makes a great, healthful appetizer when served with whole-wheat or multigrain nachos or whole-wheat toasted pita bread. I'm always asked by friends and family to bring this best-ever guacamole. If taking it to a party, you can double or triple the recipe.

Yield: 2 cups (500 mL)

> 3 ripe avocados
> 1 small tomato, chopped
> ½ small onion, diced

1 small bunch of cilantro, chopped
1 garlic clove, diced
Juice of 1 to 2 limes
Sea salt to taste

Put the avocados in a medium bowl and mash with a fork. Add the tomato, onion, cilantro, and garlic, and mix well. Stir in the lime juice, and salt to taste. Serve with multigrain tortillas or as a garnish with your favorite dish.

Hummus

Hummus makes a great appetizer or healthful snack in the middle of the day served with cut-up veggies (think bell peppers, cucumbers, and carrots) or whole-wheat pita bread, or even multigrain crackers. The chickpeas provide a nutritious source of protein, especially for your kids, who may shy away from other protein sources. Hummus is very easy to transport and make a great lunch-box item.

Yield: 4 cups (1 L)

1 (19-ounce / 540 mL) can organic chickpeas, drained and
    rinsed, reserving the liquid
½ cup (125 mL) tahini (ground sesame seeds)
3 medium garlic cloves
Dash of tamari (organic soy sauce)
Juice of 2 lemons
1½ teaspoons (7.5 mL) sea salt
Lots of black pepper
Lots of cayenne
1 teaspoon (5 mL) extra virgin olive oil or organic flaxseed oil

Put the chickpeas, tahini, garlic, tamari, lemon juice, salt, pepper, and cayenne in a food processor, and blend until smooth. If the hummus is too thick, add liquid from the chickpeas. Taste and add more lemon juice, salt, pepper, and/or cayenne as desired. Add the olive or flaxseed oil near the end to add to the creaminess. Enjoy!

Tzatziki

Tzatziki is great served with cut-up veggies (grilled or raw), chicken, lamb, or toasted pita bread. When made with Greek yogurt, it provides much more protein. The trick is to not eat the entire bowl!

Yield: 1½ cups (375 mL)

> 1 cup (250 mL) plain Greek yogurt (10% milk fat)
>   (I love the Olympic Krema brand)
> ½ cucumber, peeled and diced
> 1 to 2 garlic cloves, minced
> 1 lemon, juiced
> 1 teaspoon (5 mL) grated lemon rind
> Pinch of sea salt

Combine all the ingredients in a medium glass mixing bowl, and mix well. Adjust to taste with lemon juice and salt. Cover and refrigerate for at least 1 hour before serving.

Yummy Fruit Dip

On a special occasion, serve up this yummy dip, or keep it in an air-tight container in your refrigerator to enjoy with cut-up fruit as a snack. My nieces and nephews love this dip, and before I know it, the fruit platter is always empty.

Yield: 1½ cups (375 mL)

1 cup (250 mL) plain Greek yogurt (10% milk fat)
(I love the Olympic Krema brand)

1 single-serve (3.4-ounce / 96 g) box Jell-O vanilla instant
pudding (this is one of the few times I use a packaged
food item)

¼ cup (60 mL) whole milk

3 tablespoons (45 mL) freshly squeezed lemon juice

1 teaspoon (5 mL) grated lemon rind

Combine all the ingredients in a large mixing bowl and mix well. Serve with fresh fruit such as strawberries, raspberries, blueberries, cantaloupe, melon, bananas, and mangos.

Halibut with Mango and Goat Cheese

One of my favorite times of the year is spring, especially for all the fresh-caught fish, such as halibut and salmon. One of the best parts of living on the west coast is having access to such amazing freshly caught fish and seafood and local produce. This recipe is a huge hit with guests and one that we make often at home. The kids love the variety of flavors with the sweet from the mango and the halibut.

Yield: 4 servings

1 cup (250 mL) chopped fresh mango

2 tablespoons (30 mL) chopped Italian parsley

2 tablespoons (30 mL) freshly squeezed lime juice

½ cup (125 mL) organic maple syrup

2 tablespoons (30 mL) Dijon mustard

1 teaspoon (5 mL) coconut oil

2 tablespoons (30 mL) finely chopped leeks

Coconut or grapeseed oil for greasing

4 (4-ounce / 125 g) halibut fillets
Sea salt
¼ cup (60 mL) crumbled goat cheese

In a small bowl, combine the mango, parsley, and lime juice. Cover and refrigerate until ready to serve.

In a small saucepan over medium heat, combine the maple syrup and mustard and bring to a boil. Reduce the heat to low and simmer for 5 minutes. Remove from the heat and let cool.

Heat the 1 tablespoon (15 mL) of coconut oil in a small skillet over medium heat. Add the leeks and lightly sauté until tender. Set aside and keep warm.

Meanwhile, coat a grill rack with coconut or grapeseed oil. Preheat the grill to medium.

Season the halibut fillets with salt. Brush the fillets with the maple syrup mixture, and place them on the preheated grill. Cover and grill for 5 minutes per side, or until the fish flakes easily with a fork.

Just before serving, stir the goat cheese into the mango mixture, spoon it over the fillets, and sprinkle the cooked leeks overtop.

Halibut Italian-style

My husband, Gaetano, was born and raised in the south of Italy until he was eight years old. His mom is the best cook I know, and of course, no one in our family can ever create her version of veal, eggplant Parmesan, tomato sauce, or anything else. However, Gaetano also has a great sense of what works well together. We both love our time together in the kitchen, especially on the weekends, when we have a little more time and can relax with a glass of red wine while prepping. This recipe has recently become one of our favorite ways to prepare halibut. Purchase fresh halibut if possible, if not, then frozen will definitely work (thaw it in the fridge for 4 hours before preparing).

Yield: 4 servings

   1 (1-pound / 500 g) fresh skinless halibut fillet
   2 teaspoons (10 mL) sea salt
   Cracked black pepper to taste
   2 tablespoons (30 mL) butter, divided
   2 tablespoons (30 mL) water
   2 garlic cloves, thinly sliced
   2 cups (500 mL) halved multicolored cherry
       tomatoes, divided
   ¼ cup of white wine (optional)

Wash the halibut and pat it dry. Cover both sides with the salt and pepper. Melt 1 tablespoon (15 mL) of the butter in a medium skillet over medium heat, add the 2 tablespoons (30 mL) of water (to create a steaming effect). Add the garlic and cook for 2 minutes before adding the fish. Add the halibut and squeeze 1 cup (250 mL) of the tomatoes with your fingers (to allow the juices to separate) over the fish. Add the remaining 1 cup (250 mL) of the tomatoes to the pan along with the white wine. Cover the skillet and cook for 5 minutes. Flip the halibut, add the remaining 1 tablespoon (15 mL) of butter to the skillet, and stir the remaining 1 cup (250 mL) of tomatoes in the butter, scooping them over the fish while it cooks for another 5 minutes. This halibut is full of flavor and delicious served on a bed of quinoa with a nice green salad.

Basil Spring Salmon

Spring is an amazing time of year on the west coast, especially for the fresh-caught wild salmon. We love all types of salmon, but find the spring salmon works well for this recipe. Serve with broccolini and a spinach salad for a delicious dinner.

Yield: 4 servings

> 4 (¼-pound / 125 g) fresh spring salmon fillets (skin-on)
> 2 tablespoons (30 mL) extra virgin olive oil, divided
> 2 teaspoons (10 mL) sea salt
> Cracked black pepper, as much or as little as you like
> 1 tablespoon (15 mL) butter
> 1 garlic clove, thinly sliced
> Fresh basil, as much as you like, divided
> ¼ cup (60 mL) dry white wine

Wash and dry the salmon fillets. Cover with 1 tablespoon (15 mL) of the olive oil and the salt and pepper.

Melt the butter in a medium skillet over low heat (do not overheat the pan, otherwise the butter will burn). Add the garlic and cook for 2 minutes. Add the salmon and cover with half the basil leaves. Add the wine, cover, and steam for 5 minutes, and then flip the salmon and remove the skin (it should easily come off at this point). Cover with the remaining basil, and spoon the white wine and butter mixture overtop. Cover and cook for another 5 minutes. Serve immediately.

Curried Salmon Pasta Salad

This is a delicious salad, combining fibrous carbohydrates and healthful fats, and it is rich in protein. Make this dish for dinner, and have the leftovers for lunch the next day.

Yield: 4 servings

Salad:

  1 cup (250 mL) whole-wheat macaroni

  8 ounces (250 g) canned salmon (or possibly leftover
  salmon from dinner the night before)

  ½ cup (125 mL) minced red or yellow onion

  1 cup (250 mL) diced celery

  1 medium to large red apple, diced

  ½ cup (125 mL) chopped walnuts

Dressing:

  6 ounces (175 g) plain Greek yogurt (¾ cup / 180 mL)

  2 tablespoons (30 mL) organic flaxseed oil

  2 teaspoons (10 mL) freshly squeezed lemon juice

  2 garlic cloves, crushed

  1 teaspoon (5 mL) Dijon mustard

  ½ teaspoon (2.5 mL) salt, or to taste

  Freshly ground black pepper to taste

To make the pasta salad, cook the pasta according to the package directions; drain and rinse. In a large bowl, combine the cooked macaroni, the salmon, onion, celery, apple, and walnuts.

To make the dressing, combine all of the dressing ingredients in a small bowl and mix well. Pour the dressing over the salad and toss. Refrigerate or serve at room temperature.

Grilled Greek Chicken

This is an absolute summertime favorite with our family and with guests. It is a very simple, quick-and-easy recipe that tastes delicious. Serve with a Greek salad for a delicious "Greek-inspired" feast.

Yield: 3 servings

> 6 boneless, skinless chicken thighs
> ½ cup (125 mL) extra virgin olive oil
> ¼ cup (60 mL) tamari
> 3 tablespoons (45 mL) store-bought Greek seasoning
> (if possible, find an organic, MSG-free version)

Wash the chicken thighs and pat dry. Place the chicken in a large Ziploc bag. Add the olive oil and coat the chicken. Add the tamari and Greek seasoning. Seal the bag and marinate in the refrigerator for at least 30 minutes.

Grill on a barbecue (or bake in the oven at 350°F [180°C] for 25 to 35 minutes) until the chicken is completely cooked. The best way to grill chicken thighs is to continually turn them on the barbecue.

Grilled Greek Lamb

We are lucky to have Greek friends who have shared a few of their tried-and-true recipes. There are many things the Greeks do well, but lamb has to be one of my favorites. This is certainly a treat, and probably my favorite meat dish. Serve with grilled vegetables such as bell peppers, zucchini, red onion, and fennel. Amazing!

Yield: 2 to 3 servings

> 1 rack of lamb (fresh is best), about 8 chops
> 2 teaspoons (10 mL) sea salt
> Cracked black pepper to taste
> ½ cup (125 mL) extra virgin olive oil
> 1 to 2 garlic cloves, crushed
> Freshly squeezed lemon juice to taste
> 1 tablespoon (15 mL) dried oregano

Wash and dry the rack of lamb, and then cut it into chops and remove the excess fat. Sprinkle with the salt and pepper.

To make the marinade, combine the olive oil, garlic, lemon juice, and oregano in a bowl. Mix well.

Place the chops in the marinade, and marinate for at least 1 hour (the longer it marinates the more flavor it has).

Preheat the grill to high, and grill the chops for 6 to 7 minutes on each side. The best way to barbecue is to first sear the chops on one side, and then flip them and grill for 6 to 7 minutes, and then flip again and grill the other side for another 6 to 7 minutes. Lamb is best served medium-rare.

Variation: This recipe can also be made with rosemary and white wine. Simply substitute white wine for the lemon juice and rosemary for the oregano.

I hope you have enjoyed this small sampling of some of my favorite full-fat recipes. For more delicious, healthful recipes, please find them in *The Full-Fat Solution Recipe Book*, which is available on The Full-Fat Solution website (please visit www.thefullfatsolution.com for more information).

References

Chapter 1

1   Marjolein Bonthuis, Maria C. Hughes, Torukiri I. Ibiebele, Adèle C. Green, and Joleike C. van der Pols, "Dairy Consumption and Patterns of Mortality of Australian Adults," *European Journal of Clinical Nutrition* 64 (June 2010): 569–577.

2   Dariush Mozaffarian, Haiming Cao, Irena B. King, et al., "Trans-Palmitoleic Acid, Metabolic Risk Factors, and New-Onset Diabetes in U.S. Adults: A Cohort Study," *Annals of Internal Medicine* 153 (December 2010): 790–799.

3   Paula R. Trumbo, Sandra Schlicker, Alison A. Yates, and Mary Poos, Food and Nutrition Board of the Institute of Medicine, The National Academies, "Dietary Reference Intakes for Energy, Carbohydrate, Fiber, Fat, Fatty Acids, Cholesterol, Protein, and Amino Acids," *Journal of the American Dietetic Association* 102 (November 2002): 1621–1630.

4   No authors listed, "Trying Times for Painkiller Choices. Vioxx, Bextra, and Celebrex Can Increase the Risk for Heart Attack and Other Cardiovascular Problems. So Can the Old Standbys, Like Ibuprofen and Acetaminophen," *Harvard Heart Letter* 17 (October 2006): 1–3.

5   Charles N. Serhan, Song Hong, Karsten Gronert, et al., "Resolvins: A Family of Bioactive Products of Omega-3

Fatty Acid Transformation Circuits Initiated by Aspirin Treatment that Counter Proinflammation Signals," *Journal of Experimental Medicine* 196 (October 2002): 1025–1037.

Chapter 2

1 Victor L. Fulgoni III, Debra R. Keast, Nancy Auestad, and Erin E. Quann, "Nutrients from Dairy Foods Are Difficult to Replace in Diets of Americans: Food Pattern Modeling and an Analyses of the National Health and Nutrition Examination Survey 2003–2006," *Nutrition Research* 31 (October 2011): 759–765.

2 National Dairy Council, "Dairy Foods: A Major Nutrient Contributor to Americans' Diets," *Dairy Council Digest* 82 (September/October 2011): 33–40.

3 U.S. Department of Agriculture and U.S. Department of Health and Human Services, *Dietary Guidelines for Americans, 2010*, 7th edition (Washington, DC: U.S. Government Printing Office, December 2010), 38.

4 Amin S. Abargouei, Mohsen Janghorbani, Mohammad Salehi-Marzijarani, and Ahmad Esmaillzadeh, "Effect of Dairy Consumption on Weight and Body Composition in Adults: A Systematic Review and Meta-analysis of Randomized Controlled Clinical Trials," *International Journal of Obesity* (January 17, 2012), doi:10.1038/ijo.2011.269.

5 Patty W. Siri-Tarino, Qi Sun, Frank B. Hu, and Ronald M. Krauss, "Meta-analysis of Prospective Cohort Studies Evaluating the Association of Saturated Fat with

Cardiovascular Disease," *American Journal of Clinical Nutrition* 91 (March 2010): 535–546.

6   Chris Kresser, "Vitamin K2: The Missing Nutrient," May 6, 2008, accessed April 14, 2012, http://chriskresser.com/vitamin-k2-the-missing-nutrient.

7   Eva Warensjö, Jan-Håken Jansson, Tommy Cederholm, et al., "Biomarkers of Milk Fat and the Risk of Myocardial Infarction in Men and Women: A Prospective, Matched Case-Control Study," *American Journal of Clinical Nutrition* 92 (July 2010): 194–202.

8   Dariush Mozaffarian, Haiming Cao, Irena B. King, et al., "Circulating Palmitoleic Acid and Risk of Metabolic Abnormalities and New-Onset Diabetes," *American Journal of Clinical Nutrition* 92 (December 2010): 1350–1358.

9   Jorge E. Chavarro, Janet W. Rich-Edwards, Bernard A. Rosner, Walter C. Willet, "A Prospective Study of Dairy Foods Intake and Anovulatory Infertility," *Human Reproduction* 22 (May 2007): 1340–1347.

Chapter 3

1   Deirdre Ní Eidhin and David O'Beirne, "Oxidative Stability of Camelina Oil in Salad Dressings, Mayonnaises and during Frying," *International Journal of Food Science & Technology* 45 (March 2010): 444–452.

2   John T. Budin, William M. Breene, and Daniel H. Putnam, "Some Compositional Properties of Camelina Seeds and Oils," *Journal of the American Oil Chemists' Society* 72 (March 1995): 309–315.

3   Josef Zubr, "Oil-Seed Crop: *Camelina sativa*," *Industrial Crops and Products* 6 (February 1997): 113–119.

4   Josef Zubr, "Unique Dietary Oil from *Camelina sativa* Seed," *AgroFood Industry Hi-Tech* 20 (July–August 2009): 42–46.

5   Josef Zubr and B. Matthaus, "Effects of Growth Conditions on Fatty Acids and Tocopherols in *Camelina sativa* Oil," *Industrial Crops and Products* 15 (March 2002): 155–162.

6   Carrie H. Ruxton, Stephen C. Reed, Michael J. Simpson, and K. J. Millington, "The Health Benefits of Omega-3 Polyunsaturated Fatty Acids: A Review of the Evidence," *Journal of Human Nutrition and Dietetics* 17 (October 2004): 449–459.

7   Guixiang Zhao, Terry D. Etherton, Keith R. Martin, Shiela G. West, Peter J. Gillies, and Penny M. Kris-Etherton, "Dietary-Linolenic Acid Reduces Inflammatory and Lipid Cardiovascular Risk Factors in Hypercholesterolemic Men and Women," *Journal of Nutrition*, 134 (November 2004): 2991–2997.

8   Deirdre Ní Eidhin, Jim Burke, Brendan Lynch, and David O'Beirne, "Effects of Dietary Supplementation with Camelina Oil on Porcine Blood Lipids," *Journal of Food Science*, 68 (March 2003): 671–679.

9   Lakmali D. Amarasiri and Asoka S. Dissanayake, "Coconut Fats," *Ceylon Medical Journal* 51 (June 2006): 47–51.

10 Alan B. Feranil, Paulito L. Duazo, Christopher W. Kuzawa, and Linda S. Adair, "Coconut Oil Is Associated with a Beneficial Lipid Profile in Pre-menopausal

Women in the Philippines," *Asia Pacific Journal of Clinical Nutrition* 20 (February 2011): 190–195.

Chapter 4

1   Adam G. Tsai and Thomas A. Wadden, "Systematic Review: An Evaluation of Major Commercial Weight-Loss Programs in the United States," *Annals of Internal Medicine* 142 (January 2005): 56–66.

2   World Health Organization (WHO), "Obesity and Overweight: Fact Sheet no. 311," May 2012, accessed May 28, 2012, http://www.who.int/mediacentre/factsheets/fs311/en/index.html.

3   National Institute of Diabetes and Digestive and Kidney Diseases (NIDDK), U.S. Department of Health and Human Services, "Overweight and Obesity Statistics," National Institutes of Health (NIH) publication, updated February 2010, accessed May 28, 2012, http://win.niddk.nih.gov/publications/PDFs/stat904z.pdf.

4   Alison M. Hill, Jonathan D. Buckley, Karen J. Murphy, and Peter R. Howe, "Combining Fish-Oil Supplements with Regular Aerobic Exercise Improves Body Composition and Cardiovascular Disease Risk Factors," *American Journal of Clinical Nutrition* 85 (May 2007): 1267–1274.

5   Dolores Parra, Alfons Ramel, Narcisa Bandarra, Mairead Kiely, J. Alfredo Martínez, and Inga Thorsdottir, "A Diet Rich in Long-Chain Omega-3 Fatty Acids Modulates Satiety in Overweight and Obese Volunteers During Weight Loss, *Appetite* 51 (November 2008): 676–680.

6   M. Afzal Mir, Bambos M. Charalambous, Kevin Morgan, and P. J. Evans, "Erythrocyte Sodium Potassium-ATPase Transport in Obesity," *New England Journal of Medicine* 305 (November 1981): 1264–1268.

7   Krishna S. Vaddadi and David F. Horrobin, "Weight Loss Produced by Evening Primrose Oil Administration in Normal and Schizophrenic Individuals," *IRCS Journal of Medical Science* 7 (1979): 52–55.

8   M. Afzal Mir, Bambos M. Charalambous, Kevin Morgan, and P. J. Evans, "Erythrocyte Sodium Potassium-ATPase Transport in Obesity," *New England Journal of Medicine* 305 (November 1981): 1264–1268.

9   Stephen D. Phinney, Anna B. Tang, Debbie C. Thurmond, Manabu T. Nakamura, and Judith S. Stern, "Abnormal Polyunsaturated Lipid Metabolism in the Obese Zucker Rat, with Partial Metabolic Correction by Gamma-Linolenic Acid Administration," *Metabolism* 42 (September 1993): 1127–1140.

10 Ryozo Takada, Mamoru Saitoh, and Tom Mori, "Dietary Gamma-Linolenic Acid-Enriched Oil Reduces Body Fat Content and Induces Liver Enzyme Activities Relating to Fatty Acid Beta-Oxidation in Rats," *Journal of Nutrition* 124 (April 1994): 469–474.

11 Marie A. Schirmer and Stephen D. Phinney, "-Linolenate Reduces Weight Regain in Formerly Obese Humans," *Journal of Nutrition* 137 (June 2007): 1430–1435.

12 Leigh E. Norris, Angela L. Collene, Michelle L. Asp, et al., "Comparison of Dietary Conjugated Linoleic Acid with Safflower Oil on Body Composition in Obese Postmenopausal Women with Type-2 Diabetes Mellitus,"

American Journal of Clinical Nutrition 90 (September 2009): 468–476.

13 M. L. Assunção, H. S. Ferreira, A. F. dos Santos, C. R. Cabral Jr., and T. M. Florêncio, "Effects of Dietary Coconut Oil on the Biochemical and Antropometric Profiles of Women Presenting Abdominal Obesity," *Lipids* 44 (July 2009): 593–601.

14 Jo Robinson, *Why Grassfed Is Best* (Vashon, WA: Vashon Island Press, 2000).

15 Jess Halliday, NutraIngredients.com, "CLA's Body-Shaping Action Clarified in New Trial," May 10, 2006, accessed May 28, 2012, http://www.nutraingredients.com/Research/CLA-s-body-shaping-action-clarified-in-new-trial.

16 Erling Thom, Jan Wadstein, and Ola Gudmundsen, "Conjugated Linoleic Acid Reduces Body Fat in Healthy Exercising Humans," *Journal of International Medicine Research* 29 (May 2001): 392–396.

17 Leila Azadbakht, Parvin Mirmiran, Ahmad Esmaillzadeh, and Fereidoun Azizi, "Dairy Consumption Is Inversely Associated with the Prevalence of the Metabolic Syndrome in Tehranian Adults," *American Journal of Clinical Nutrition* 82 (September 2005): 523–530.

Chapter 5

1 Alan S. Ryan, James D. Astwood, Sheila Gautier, Connye N. Kuratko, Edward B. Nelson, and Norman Salem Jr., "Effects of Long-Chain Polyunsaturated Fatty Acid Supplementation on Neurodevelopment

in Childhood: A Review of Human Studies," *Prostaglandins, Leukotrienes & Essential Fatty Acids* 82 (April–June 2010): 305–314.

2 Colette Montgomery, Brian K. Speake, Alan Cameron, Naveed Sattar, and Lawrence T. Weaver, "Maternal Docosahexaenoic Acid Supplementation and Fetal Accretion," *British Journal of Nutrition* 90 (July 2003): 135–143.

3 Gregory J. Anderson, William E. Connor, and Julie D. Corliss, "Docosahexaenoic Acid Is the Preferred Dietary n-3 Fatty Acid for the Development of the Brain and Retina," *Pediatric Research* 27 (January 1990): 89–97.

4 Sjúrður F. Olsen, Jannie D. Sørensen, Niels J. Secher, et al., "Randomised Controlled Trial of Effect of Fish-Oil Supplementation on Pregnancy Duration," *Lancet* 339 (April 1992): 1003–1007.

5 James A. Greenberg, Stacey J. Bell, and Wendy Van Ausdal, "Omega-3 Fatty Acid Supplementation During Pregnancy," *Obstetrics & Gynecology* 1 (Fall 2008): 162–169.

6 Sjúrður F. Olsen and Niels J. Secher, "Low Consumption of Seafood in Early Pregnancy as a Risk Factor for Preterm Delivery: Prospective Cohort Study," *British Medical Journal* 324 (February 2002): 447–450.

7 US Environmental Protection Agency, "The Effects of Heavy Metal Exposures during Pregnancy on Maternal and Infant Health," May 2009, accessed June 4, 2012, http://cfpub.epa.gov/ncer_abstracts/index.cfm/fuseaction/display.abstractDetail/abstract/8196/report/0.

8   U.S. Food and Drug Administration, Federal Register, Department of Health & Human Services, "Report of Quantitative Risk and Benefit Assessment of Commercial Fish Consumption, Focusing on Neurodevelopment Effects (Measured by Verbal Development in Children) and on Coronary Heart Disease and Stroke in the General Population, and Summary of Published Research on the Beneficial Effects of Fish Consumption and Omega-3 Fatty Acids for Certain Neurodevelopmental and Cardiovascular Endpoints," January 21, 2009, accessed May 31, 2012, http://www.fda.gov/Food/FoodSafety/Product-SpecificInformation/Seafood/FoodbornePathogensContaminants/Methylmercury/ucm088765.htm.

9   Institute of Medicine, "Seafood Choices: Balancing Benefits and Risks," October 2006, accessed May 31, 2012, http://www.iom.edu/~/media/Files/Report%20Files/2006/Seafood-Choices-Balancing-Benefits-and-Risks/11762_SeafoodChoicesReportBrief.pdf.

10 US Department of Health and Human Services, US Department of Agriculture, "Dietary Guidelines for Americans 2005," accessed June 1, 2012, http://www.health.gov/dietaryguidelines/dga2005/document/pdf/DGA2005.pdf.

11 US Department of Agriculture, Agricultural Research Service, National Agricultural Library, "USDA National Nutrient Database for Standard Reference," December 2011, accessed June 1, 2012, http://ndb.nal.usda.gov/.

12 Association of Reproductive Health Professionals, "Fish Consumption to Promote Good Health and Minimize Contaminants," September 2008, accessed June 1, 2012,

http://www.arhp.org/publications-and-resources/quick-reference-guide-for-clinicians/fish-and-health/summary.

13 Michelle P. Judge, Ofel Harel, and Carol J. Lammi-Keefe, "A Docosahexaenoic Acid–Functional Food during Pregnancy Benefits Infant Visual Acuity at Four but Not Six Months of Age. *Lipids* 42 (March 2007): 117–122.

14 Eileen E. Birch, Sharon Garfield, Dennis R. Hoffman, Ricardo Uauy, and David G. Birch, "A Randomized Controlled Trial of Early Dietary Supply of Long-Chain Polyunsaturated Fatty Acids and Mental Development in Term Infants," *Developmental Medicine and Child Neurology* 42 (March 2000): 174–181.

15 Sunita R. Cheruku, Hawley E. Montgomery-Downs, Susanna L. Farkas, Evelyn B. Thoman, and Carol J. Lammi-Keefe, "Higher Maternal Plasma Docosahexaenoic Acid during Pregnancy Is Associated with More Mature Neonatal Sleep-State Patterning," *American Journal of Clinical Nutrition* 76 (September 2002): 608–613.

16 Michael T. Clandinin, Janet E. Chappell, Tibor Heim, Paul R. Swyer, and Graham W. Chance, "Fatty Acid Utilization in Perinatal de Novo Synthesis of Tissues," *Early Human Development* 5 (September 1981): 355–366.

17 James R. Drover, Dennis R. Hoffman, Yolanda S. Casteñeda, et al., "Cognitive Function in 18-Month-Old Term Infants of the DIAMOND Study: A Randomized, Controlled Clinical Trial with Multiple Dietary Levels of Docosahexaenoic Acid," *Early Human Development* 87 (March 2011): 223–230.

18 Ingrid B. Helland, Ola D. Suagstad, Kristin Saarem, Adriana C. van Houwelingen, Gro Nylander, and Christian A. Drevon, "Supplementation of n-3 Fatty Acids during Pregnancy and Lactation Reduces Maternal Plasma Lipid Levels and Provides DHA to the Infants," *Journal of Maternal-Fetal and Neonatal Medicine* 19 (July 2006): 397–406.

19 Janet A. Dunstan, Trevor A. Mori, Anne E. Barden, et al., "Effects of n-3 Polyunsaturated Fatty Acid Supplementation in Pregnancy on Maternal and Fetal Erythrocyte Fatty Acid Composition," *European Journal of Clinical Nutrition* 59 (March 2004): 429–437.

20 Cornelius M. Smuts, Minzhao Huang, David Mundy, Terry Plasse, Stacey Major, and Susan E. Carlson, "A Randomized Trial of Docosahexaenoic Acid Supplementation during the Third Trimester of Pregnancy," *Obstetrics & Gynecology* 101 (March 2003): 469–479.

21 M. Victoria Escolano-Margarit, Rosa Ramos, Jeannette Beyer, et al., "Prenatal DHA Status and Neurological Outcome in Children at Age 5.5 Years Are Positively Associated," *Journal of Nutrition* 141 (June 2011): 1216–1223.

22 Maria Makrides and Robert A. Gibson, "Long-Chain Polyunsaturated Fatty Acid Requirements during Pregnancy and Lactation," *American Journal of Clinical Nutrition* 71 (January 2000): 307S–311S.

23 Arild E. Hansen, Hilda F. Wiese, Arr Nell Boelsche, Mary Ellen Haggard, Doris J. D. Adam, and Helen Davis, "Role of Linoleic Acid in Infant Nutrition: Clinical and Chemical Study of 428 Infants on Milk

Mixtures Varying in Kind and Amount of Fat," *Pediatrics* 31 (January 1963): 171–192.

24 Colette Montgomery, Brian K. Speake, Alan Cameron, Naveed Sattar, and Lawrence T. Weaver, "Maternal Docosahexaenoic Acid Supplementation and Fetal Accretion," *British Journal of Nutrition* 90 (July 2003): 135–143.

25 Robin G. Jordan, "Prenatal Omega-3 Fatty Acids: Review and Recommendations," *Journal of Midwifery & Women's Health*, 55 (November 2010): 520–528.

26 Emma Goksör, Bernt Alm, Hrefna Thengilsdottir, Rolf Pettersson, Nils Åberg, and Göran G. Wennergren, "Preschool Wheeze—Impact of Early Fish Introduction and Neonatal Antibiotics," *Acta Paediatrica* 100 (December 2011): 1561–1566.

27 Ibid.

28 Larry B. Silver, "Attention-Deficit/Hyperactivity Disorder in Adult Life," *Child and Adolescent Psychiatry Clinics of North America* 9 (July 2000): 511–523.

29 Larry Scahill and Mary Schwab-Stone, "Epidemiology of ADHD in School-Age Children," *Child and Adolescent Psychiatry Clinics of North America* 9 (July 2000): 541–555.

30 Jan Philippe Schuchardt, Michael Huss, Manuela Stauss-Grabo, and Andreas Hahn, "Significance of Long-Chain Polyunsaturated Fatty Acids (PUFAs) for the Development and Behavior of Children," *European Journal of Pediatrics* 169 (February 2010): 149–164.

31 Arild E. Hansen, Hilda F. Wiese, Arr Nell Boelsche, Mary Ellen Haggard, Doris J. D. Adam, and Helen Davis, "Role of Linoleic Acid in Infant Nutrition: Clinical and Chemical Study of 428 Infants on Milk Mixtures Varying in Kind and Amount of Fat," *Pediatrics* 31 (January 1963): 171–192.

32 Laura J. Stevens, Sydney S. Zentall, John L. Deck, et al., "Essential Fatty Acid Metabolism in Boys with Attention-Hyperactivity Disorder," *American Journal of Clinical Nutrition* 62 (October 1995): 233–239.

33 Rebecca Knickmeyer, Simon Baron-Cohen, Peter Raggatt, and Kevin Taylor, "Foetal Testosterone, Social Relationships, and Restricted Interests in Children," *Journal of Child Psychology and Psychiatry* 46 (February 2005): 198–210.

34 Alexandra J. Richardson and Basant K. Puri, "A Randomized Double-Blind, Placebo-Controlled Study of the Effects of Supplementation with Highly Unsaturated Fatty Acids on ADHD-Related Symptoms in Children with Specific Learning Difficulties," *Progress in Neuropsychopharmacology and Biological Psychiatry* 26 (February 2002): 233–239.

35 Jacqueline Stordy, "Essential Fatty Acids (EFAs) and Learning Disorders," *Holistic Health Journal* 4 (October 1997).

36 Alexandra J. Richardson and Basant K. Puri, "The Potential Role of Fatty Acids in Attention-Deficit/ Hyperactivity Disorder," *Prostaglandins, Leukotrienes & Essential Fatty Acids* 63 (July–August 2000): 79–87.

37 Alexandra J. Richardson and Paul Montgomery, "The Oxford-Durham Study: A Randomized, Controlled Trial of Dietary Supplementation with Fatty Acids in Children with Developmental Coordination Disorder," *Pediatrics* 115 (May 2005): 1360–1366.

38 David J. Posey and Christopher J. McDougle, "Pharmacotherapeutic Management of Autism," *Expert Opinion in Pharmacothery* 2 (April 2001): 587–600.

39 Stephen T. Schultz, Hillary S. Klonoff-Cohen, Deborah L. Wingard, et al., "Breastfeeding, Infant Formula Supplementation, and Autistic Disorder: The Results of a Patient Survey," *International Breastfeeding Journal* 1 (September 2006): 16.

40 John Gordon Bell, Elizabeth E. MacKinlay, James R. Dick, Donald J. MacDonald, Rose M. Boyle, and Alastair C. Glen, "Essential Fatty Acids and Phopholipase A2 in Autistic Spectrum Disorders," *Prostaglandins, Leukotrienes & Essential Fatty Acids* 71 (October 2004): 201–204.

Chapter 6

1 Charles M. Alexander, Pamela B. Landsman, Steven M. Teutsch, and Steven M. Haffner, Third National Health and Nutrition Examination Survey (NHANES III); National Cholesterol Education Program (NCEP), "NCEP-Defined Metabolic Syndrome, Diabetes, and Prevalence of Coronary Heart Disease among NHANES III Participants Age 50 Years and Older," *Diabetes* 52 (May 2003): 1210–1241.

2   Ethan Watters, "DNA Is Not Destiny," *Discover Magazine* 75 (November 2006): 32–37.

3   Expert Panel on Detection, Evaluation, and Treatment of High Blood Cholesterol in Adults, "Executive Summary of the Third Report of the National Cholesterol Education Program (NCEP)," *Journal of the American Medical Association* 285 (May 2001): 2486–2497.

4   Kenji Maeda, Yoshinori Noguchi, and Tsuguya Fukui, "The Effects of Cessation from Cigarette Smoking on the Lipid and Lipoprotein Profiles: A Meta-analysis," *Preventive Medicine* 47 (October 2003): 283–290.

5   CBS News, "CDC: Only 13 Percent of Americans Have High Cholesterol," April 25, 2012, accessed June 6, 2012, http://www.cbsnews.com/8301-504763_162-57421375-10391704/cdc-only-13-percent-of-americans-have-high-cholesterol.

6   Lawrence A. Leiter, Darlene Abbott, Norman R. C. Campbell, Rena Mendelson, Richard I. Ogilvie, and Arun Chockalingam, "Recommendations on Obesity and Weight Loss," *Canadian Medical Association Journal* 160 (May 1999): S7–S12.

7   Luc Djoussé, James S. Pankow, John H. Eckfeldt, et al., "Relation between Dietary Linoleic Acid and Coronary Artery Disease in the National Heart, Lung, and Blood Institute Family Heart Study," *American Journal of Clinical Nutrition* 74 (November 2001): 612–619.

8   Frank B. Hu, Leslie Bronner, Walter C. Willett, et al., "Fish and Omega-3 Fatty Acid Intake and Risk of Coronary Heart Disease in Women," *Journal of the American Medical Association* 287 (April 2002): 1815–1821.

9 Fuxia Jin, David C. Nieman, Wei Sha, Guoxiang Xie, Yunping Qiu, and Wei Jia, "Supplementation of Milled Chia Seeds Increases Plasma ALA and EPA in Postmenopausal Women," *Plant Foods for Human Nutrition* 67 (June 2012): 105–110.

10 Martha Guevara-Cruz, Armando R. Tovar, Carlos A. Aquilar-Salinas, et al., "A Dietary Pattern Including Nopal, Chia Seed, Soy Protein, and Oat Reduces Serum Triglycerides and Glucose Intolerance in Patients with Metabolic Syndrome," *Journal of Nutrition* 142 (January 2012): 64–69.

11 Jorn Dyerberg and Hans O. Bang, "Lipid Metabolism, Atherogenesis, and Haemostasis in Eskimos: The Role of the Prostaglandin-3 Family," *Haemostasis* 8 (1979): 227–233.

12 Leo Galland, "Diet and Inflammation," *Nutrition in Clinical Practice* 25 (December 2010): 634–640.

13 Paul M. Ridker, "Clinical Application of C-Reactive Protein for Cardiovascular Disease Detection and Prevention," *Circulation* 107 (January 2003): 363–398.

14 Mahmoud Ebrahimi, Majid Ghayour-Mobarhan, Samaneh Rezaiean, et al., "Omega-3 Fatty Acid Supplements Improve the Cardiovascular Risk Profile of Subjects with Metabolic Syndrome, Including Markers of Inflammation and Auto-immunity," *Acta Cardiologica* 64 (June 2009): 321–327.

15 William S. Harris, "n-3 Fatty Acids and Serum Lipoproteins: Human Studies," *American Journal of Clinical Nutrition* 65 (March 1997): 1645S–1654S.

16 Harold E. Bays, Ann P. Tighe, Richard Sadovsky, and
    Michael H. Davidson, "Prescription Omega-3 Fatty Acids
    and Their Lipid Effects: Physiological Mechanisms of
    Action and Their Clinical Implications," *Expert Review of
    Cardiovascular Therapy* 6 (March 2008): 391–409.

17 William S. Harris, Henry N. Ginsberg, Narin Arunakul,
    et al., "Safety and Efficacy of Omacor in Severe
    Hypertriglyceridemia," *Journal of Cardiovascular Risk* 4
    (October–December 1997): 385–391.

18 Michael H. Davidson, Evan A. Stein, Harold E. Bayes, et
    al., for the COMBination of prescription Omega-3 with
    Simvastatin (COMBOS) Investigators, "Efficacy and
    Tolerability of Adding Prescription Omega-3 Fatty Acids
    4 g/d to Simvastatin 40 mg/d in Hypertriglyceridemic
    Patients: An 8-week, Randomized, Double-Blind,
    Placebo-Controlled Study," *Clinical Therapeutics* 29
    (July 2007): 1354–1367.

19 Gerd Assman and Helmut Schulte, "Relation of High-
    Density Lipoprotein Cholesterol and Triglycerides to
    Incidence of Atherosclerotic Coronary Artery Disease
    (the PROCAM Experience). Prospective Cardiovascular
    Munster Study," *American Journal of Cardiology* 70
    (September 1992): 733–737.

20 Boli Huang, Pengfei Wu, Melissa M. Bowker-Kinley, and
    Robert A. Harris, "Regulation of Pyruvate Dehydrogenase
    Kinase Expression by Peroxisome Proliferator-Activated
    Receptor-alpha Ligands, Glucocorticoids, and Insulin,"
    Diabetes 51 (February 2002): 276–283.

21 Alexander Leaf, Jing X. Kang, Yong-Fu Xiao, and
    George E. Billman, "Clinical Prevention of Sudden

Cardiac Death by n-3 Polyunsaturated Fatty Acids and Mechanism of Prevention of Arrhythmias by n-3 Fish Oils," *Circulation* 107 (June 2003): 2646–2652.

22 Rishi G. Anand, Mohi Alkadri, Carl J. Lavie, and Richard V. Milani, "The Role of Fish Oil in Arrhythmia Prevention," *Journal of Cardiopulmonary Rehabilitation and Prevention* 28 (March 2008): 92–98.

23 Dariush Mozaffarian, Ronald J. Prineas, Phyllis K. Stein, and David S. Siscovick, "Dietary Fish and n-3 Fatty Acid Intake and Cardiac Electrocardiographic Parameters in Humans," *Journal of the American College of Cardiology* 48 (August 2006): 478–484.

24 Michael L. Burr, Ann M. Fehily, J. F. Gilbert, et al., "Effects of Changes in Fat, Fish, and Fibre Intakes on Death and Myocardial Reinfarction: Diet and Reinfarction Trial (DART)," *Lancet* 2 (September 1989): 757–761.

25 No authors listed, "Dietary Supplementation with n-3 Polyunsaturated Fatty Acids and Vitamin E after Myocardial Infarction: Results of the GISSI-Prevenzione Trial. Gruppo Italiano per lo Studio della Sopravvivenza nell'Infarto Miocardico," *Lancet* 354 (August 1999): 447–455.

26 Mitsuhiro Yokoyama, Hideki Origasa, Masunori Matsuzaki, et al., "Effects of Eicosapentaenoic Acid on Major Coronary Events in Hypercholesterolaemic Patients (JELIS): A Randomized Open-Label, Blinded Endpoint Analysis," *Lancet* 369 (March 2007): 1090–1098.

27 Roxandra Bunea, Khassan El Farrah, and Luisa Deutsch, "Evaluation of the Effects of Neptune Krill Oil on the

Clinical Course of Hyperlipidemia," *Alternative Medicine Review* 9 (December 2004): 420–428.

28 American Heart Association, "Fish and Omega-3 Fatty Acids," September 2010, accessed June 6, 2012, http://www.heart.org/HEARTORG/GettingHealthy/ NutritionCenter/HealthyDietGoals/Fish-and-Omega-3-Fatty-Acids_UCM_303248_Article.jsp.

Chapter 7

1 Ronald A. Hites, Jeffery A. Foran, David O. Carpenter, M. Coreen Hamilton, Barbara A. Knuth, and Steven J. Schwager, "Global Assessment of Organic Contaminants in Farmed Salmon," *Science* 303 (January 2004): 226–229.

2 Walter J. Crinnion, "The Role of Persistent Organic Pollutants in the Worldwide Epidemic of Type-2 Diabetes Mellitus and the Possible Connection to Farmed Atlantic Salmon (*Salmo salar*)," *Alternative Medicine Review* 16 (December 2011): 301–313.

3 Wikipedia, "Fish Farming," last modified May 24, 2012, accessed June 6, 2012, http://en.wikipedia.org/wiki/ Fish_farming.

4 Susan Schwartz, "The Oils in Fish Are Good for Us, but the Accumulated Pollutants Are Not. A Blogger Tells Us How to Stay in the Pink," *The Vancouver Sun*, May 3, 2012, http://www.vancouversun.com/life/green-guide/ down+dirty+salmon/6559229/story.html.

Recommended Reading

Chilton, Floyd H. *Inflammation Nation: The First Clinically Proven Eating Plan to End Our Nation's Secret Epidemic.* New York: Fireside, 2005.

Daniel, Kaayla T. *The Whole Soy Story: The Dark Side of America's Favorite Health Food.* Washington, DC: New Trends Publishing, 2005.

Enig, Mary G. *Know Your Fats: The Complete Primer for Understanding the Nutrition of Fats, Oils, and Cholesterol.* Silver Spring, MD: Bethesda Press, 2000.

Erasmus, Udo. *Fats That Heal, Fats That Kill.* Burnaby, BC: Alive Books, 1993.

Fife, Bruce. *The Coconut Oil Miracle.* New York: Penguin Group, 2004.

Gittleman, Ann Louise. *The Fat Flush Plan.* New York: McGraw Hill, 2001.

———. *The Fat Flush Cookbook.* New York: McGraw Hill, 2003.

Joiner-Bey, Herb. *The Healing Power of Flax.* Los Angeles: Freedom Press, 2010.

Morello, Gaetano. *Whole Body Cleansing: Transform Your Health through Gentle Purification and Effective Detoxification.* El Segundo, CA: Active Interest Media, 2009.

Stoll, Andrew. *The Omega-3 Connection.* New York: Simon & Schuster, 2002.

Resources

Recommended Health and Nutrition Brand

GAB Innovations Inc.
Sea-licious®
7860 Venture Street
Burnaby, BC
V5A 1V3
www.sea-licious.ca

Sea-licious is the best-tasting fish oil on the market, guaranteed. Sea-licious offers the highest quality, most pure omega oils to help your entire family achieve optimal health and wellness. Sea-licious prides itself on partnering with International Fish Oil Standards (IFOS) to verify the quality and purity of every bottle of Sea-licious. As a mother, dietitian, natural-health author, and expert on omega-3s, I believe wholeheartedly in the benefits of omega nutrition for the entire family.

Suppliers of Quality Omega-3 and Omega-6 Oils

Biodroga
301 Joseph Carrier
Vaudreuil-Dorion, QC
Canada
J7V 5V5
Toll-free: 1-800-371-9668
United States: biodrogausa.com
Canada: biodroga.ca

Biodroga specializes in the supply and product development of omega-3 and omega-6 plant- and marine-based ingredients included in many popular supplements found in health-food and drug stores today. With major developments in essential fatty acids over the last twenty-five years, it can count on an international network of advisors enabling it to bring innovative concepts to the North American nutraceutical market.

Bioriginal Food & Science
102 Melville Street
Saskatoon, SK
Canada
S7J 0R1
Phone: 1-306-975-1166
www.bioriginal.com

Bioriginal Food & Science is a global provider of innovative essential fatty acid solutions. Their products are used in nutraceuticals, functional foods, skin care products, cosmetics, animal feed, veterinary products, and over-the-counter pharmaceuticals. They have offices and facilities in Canada, the United States, Europe, and China, enabling international distribution of their innovative EFA products.

Pharmachem Laboratories
265 Harrison Avenue
Kearny, NJ
USA
07032
Phone: 1-201-246-1000
Toll-free: 1-800-526-0609
Email: info@pharmachemlabs.com
www.pharmachemlabs.com

Pharmachem Laboratories is a premier international innovator, manufacturer, and supplier of the finest-quality ingredients. They deliver optimal solutions tailored to meet consumers' needs across a complex matrix of industries, including nutritionals, food and beverages, flavors, and fragrances. Pharmachem is the exclusive distributor of Benexia (chia seed and oil) as well as Ecosea Krill Oil.

Other Recommended Nutrition and Food Brands

Raincoast Trading
Delta, BC
Canada
V4C 4R8
www.raincoasttrading.com

Raincoast Trading has been selling premium wild seafood products since 1978. Based in Vancouver on the west coast of Canada, the company is proud to offer consumers sustainably harvested gourmet canned seafood. Raincoast Trading adheres to the highest sustainability standards when catching, processing, and packaging its seafood. The company's seafood is single-cooked and packed in natural fish oils, which results in a rich, dense flavor and loads of extra nutrition typically not found in most canned seafood products.

Vitamix
Toll-free: 1-800-848-2649
www.vitamix.com

Visit the Vitamix website for live demonstrations of truly the best, most powerful blender I have ever used. I absolutely love this tool as a way to increase the fruit and vegetables in my diet. I recommend everyone to invest in a Vitamix.

Quality Assurance Testing

Nutrasource Diagnostics
International Fish Oil Standards Program
120 Research Lane, Suite 203
University of Guelph Research Park
Guelph, ON
Canada
N1G 0B4
www.ifosprogram.com

Nutrasource Diagnostics provides the International Fish Oil Standards (IFOS) Program, which is a third-party testing and accreditation program for omega-3 fish oil products.

Informational Websites

Agriculture and Agri-Food Canada (source of fish and seafood fact sheets): www.ats-sea.agr.gc.ca/sea-mer/fhs-eng.htm

Dietitians of Canada: www.dietitians.ca

Flax Council of Canada: www.flaxcouncil.ca

Karlene Karst, Registered Dietitian: www.karlenekarst.com

Lorna Vanderhaeghe, Lorna Vanderhaeghe Health Solutions: www.lornavanderhaeghe.com

PubMed (source of biomedical literature): www.ncbi.nlm.nih.gov/pubmed

The Full-Fat Solution: www.thefullfatsolution.com

Index

Note: t represents a table.

A

Asia Pacific Journal of Clinical Nutrition, 61
aspirin, 21, 133–34
astaxanthin, 31
asthma, 110–11
ATPase metabolic process, 81
attention-deficit disorder (ADD), 108, 112–13
attention-deficit hyperactive disorder (ADHD), 108, 112–13, 114–15
autism, 115–16
autoimmune diseases, 27–28
avocado oil, 56–57
avocados, 32, 157, 160–61

B

babies, 98–99, 104–8, 110–11, 118
   See also children
bananas, 155
BAT (brown adipose tissue), 81
beef, 11
behavioral problems, 112–16
belly fat, 79, 83–86
berries, 153–54, 154
beta-carotene, 31
better butter, 10, 53
blood. See cholesterol; triglycerides
blood sugar, 86–87
BMI (body mass index), 128–29
borage oil, 27–28, 82–83
brain development, 104–6
breast milk, 106–10
Brie cheese, 159
British Journal of Nutrition, 97
broccoli, 13
brown adipose tissue (BAT), 81
Brussels sprouts, 13
butter

energy, 10, 11

EPA (eicosapentaenoic acid)

    benefits of, 132–33t

    in breast milk, 107–8

    DHA (docosahexaenoic acid) and, 22–23

    dietary concerns with, 108–9

    in fish, 103t, 139–40t

    metabolism of, 22

    sources of, 33

    See also DHA (docosahexaenoic acid); omega-3 fatty acids

essential fatty acids (EFAs). See EFAs (essential fatty acids)

evening primrose oil, 13

eye development, 104, 108

F

fad diets, 73–74

fat cells, 14–16, 76

fats

    benefits of, 31–32

    importance of, 4–5

    increase in, 52–54

    metabolism of, 77

    misconceptions about, 3

    recommendations for, 90–91

    types of, 8, 37–38

    See also oils; saturated fats; trans fats; unsaturated fats

fat-soluble phytonutrients, 31

fatty acids, 12–13, 77, 97–98, 123

    See also omega-3 fatty acids; omega-6 fatty acids; polyunsaturated

        fatty acids (PUFAs)

FDA (Food & Drug Administration), 101–2, 101t

fertility, 39–40

    See also pregnancies; women

fertilizers, 25–27

Fiji Organics, 60

GISSI (Gruppo Italiano per lo Studio della Sopravvivenza nell'Infarto Miocardico)-Prevenzione study, 137
GLA (gamma-linoleic acid), 13, 25–28, 32, 53, 81–83
goat cheese, 163–64
goat's milk, 43
Goodness Me Market, 57
grains, 8, 91
grapeseed oil, 24, 62–63
Greek chicken, 167–68
Greek lamb, 168–69
Greek salad, 158
Greek yogurt, 9, 43–44, 162, 162–63
guacamole, 160–61

H
halibut, 163–64, 164–65
Harvard School of Public Health, 9
hazelnut oil, 63
HDL (high-density lipoprotein), 125–27, 128
heart attacks, 39, 136–37
heart disease
    arrhythmias and, 135–36
    dairy and, 35
    fish and, 132
    low-fat foods and, 3, 7
    obesity and, 128–29
    research on, 9, 130
    saturated fats and, 3, 9, 10–11, 38
    See also cardiovascular disease (CVD)
heart health, 137–38, 140–41
hemp milk, 42
hemp seed oil, 24, 63–64
hemp seeds, 13
Hibbeln, Joseph, 107
high-density lipoprotein (HDL), 125–27, 128
hormones, 16–17, 79–80, 84–85

preserved foods, 8

probiotics, 110

processed foods, 8

prostaglandins, 19–20, 21–22

protectins, 22–23

protein, 90, 154

PUFAs (polyunsaturated fatty acids), 12–13, 13, 33t

pumpkin seed oil, 66

purslane, 13, 48

Q

Queensland Institute of Medical Research, 9

R

red meat, 11

resolvins, 22–23

rheumatoid arthritis, 22–23

rice bran oil, 66–67

rice milk, 42

S

safflower oil, 13, 67, 83–87

salad dressings, 53, 157, 159, 160, 166–67

salads, 157, 158, 159, 166–67

salmon, 149–51, 149t, 166, 166–67

Salmon, Ruth, 149

satiety hormones, 79–80

saturated fats

    cells and, 15–16

    chronic diseases and, 38

    daily diet and, 54

    dairy and, 8–9, 34

    heart disease and, 3, 9, 10–11, 38

T

U

V

W

About the Author

Karlene Karst, RD, is a leading expert in nutrition and natural health. Karlene holds a BSc in nutrition from the University of Saskatchewan, Canada, and is a registered dietitian. Karlene is the author of several books and is a highly sought-after, enthusiastic, and passionate individual who has appeared on *QVC, Access Hollywood,* and *Canada AM.* She is a frequent guest speaker at educational events around North America. Karlene is a mom to two young boys, Luca and Matteo, and resides in beautiful Vancouver, British Columbia, Canada.

www.karlenekarst.com